# Doorways to Learning

# Doorways to Learning

## A Model for Developing the Brain's Full Potential

Peter Majoy

Zephyr Press
Tucson, Arizona

Doorways to Learning
A Model for Developing the Brain's Full Potential

Grades K–12


Printed in the United States of America

ISBN 0-913705-86-1

Editors: Stacey Lynn and Stacey Shropshire
Cover design: Nancy Taylor
Design and production: Nancy Taylor

Zephyr Press
P.O. Box 13448
Tucson, Arizona 85732-3448



Copyright Acknowledgments appear on page 236.

Library of Congress Cataloging-in-Publication Data

Majoy, Peter, 1943-
7 doorways : a model for developing the brain's full potential / Peter Majoy.
p. cm.
Includes bibliographical references.
ISBN 0-913705-86-1
1. Learning. 2. Learning—Physiological aspects. 3. Brain--Localization of function. I. Title. II. Title: Seven doorways.
LB1060.M323 1993
370. 15'23—dc20 93-8573

*The 7 Doorways model is derived from the network of neural connectivity that is innate in humans; it is a natural framework on which to build a variety of educational programs.*

# Contents

# INTRODUCTION
## Model Shifting

*Mythoscience is not necessarily understood, but the findings ring a bell. Take, for example, the Pygmalion Effect, wherein the measurable intelligence of youngsters was dramatically increased by manipulating their teachers' assumptions.*

—Marilyn Ferguson, *New Sense*

Everything we do in education is prophetic, because education creates the future. If we are sharp we can forecast the future and shape it through the things we do as teachers. Kids look into our individual and corporate eyes, gazing at our souls. They see what we think of them and the dreams we are committed to in order to bring to pass their aspirations. But it is difficult to stay committed to positive dreams for our students. Thousands of schoolteachers are confronted each year with what can only be called missionary situations. They go through an annual numbing process faced as they are with overwhelming problems, declining resources, and school systems that have lost imagination and creative spirit. Each day is merely a holding pattern of containment and burnout.

Some teachers continue to try to meet the challenges of teaching under such circumstances. Tracy Kidder (1989) tells of Chris Zajac, a real-life hero, who ends another year at the Kelly School in Holyoke, one of

Massachusetts's most underfunded, problem-riddled systems. Zajac's testimony to the undying commitment of teachers can be fished from Kidder's closing description:

> An hour later she was driving under the railroad bridge. She crossed the first canal, which marks the edge of the Flats. She probably wouldn't see this part of town again, or any of her walkers until September. Within a few weeks this year's disappointments would begin to fade. Now they were still fresh. She thought about Robert. "He's my failure, I guess. Him and Clarence." Even the most troubled children had attractive qualities for Chris. Even the most toughened, she always felt, wanted to please her and wanted her to like them, no matter how perversely they expressed it. She belonged among schoolchildren. They made her confront sorrow and injustice. They made her feel useful. Again this year, some had needed more help than she could provide. There were many problems that she hadn't solved. But it wasn't for lack of trying. She hadn't given up. She had run out of time. (331)

Zajac's commitment is beyond reproach, but teachers like her are denied the fullness of their vocation by systems that are choked either by lack of money or by fear of change. Unless we commit ourselves to a revolution in education, we are marking time we do not have to spare.

Michael Hutchinson (1986) reports on the work of Mark Rosenzweig and Marion Diamond, who claim brain cells can revive, new ones appear, and the weight and complexity of neural networks in the cerebral cortex increase if two conditions exist: challenge and relaxation. Today's schools are loci neither of challenge nor of relaxation; they have become instead havens of control of body and mind. Most of our schools are boring and have become breeding grounds for laziness; boredom and laziness retard brain growth and development. It is imperative that schools and teachers begin shifting models, downsizing, and building curriculum with the power and mandate to experiment. The 7 Doorways model aims at nothing less than challenging teachers and decision makers to fish or cut bait in the high and turbulent seas of contemporary education.

We need a model that respects individual style while calling for that style to stretch itself intentionally into other domains. We also need an integrated system. If parts of the brain are not stimulated and used, exercised and challenged, the whole brain (and the whole person) suffers. If the whole is not addressed, the parts decline in effectiveness.

Such a model should be based on a generic blueprint for learning that crosses ability groups, age groups, disciplines, and socioeconomic boundaries, reflecting an inquiry into the "inner blueprint" of which Joseph Chilton Pearce (1985) wrote. The model should be cohesive, dynamic, and open; it should provide a good basis for developing curriculum that is both challenging and conducive to relaxed awareness. Because the 7 Doorways model is derived from the network of neural connectivity that is innate in humans, it is a natural framework on which to build a variety of educational programs. We see in this model a system in which the whole is at the disposal of its parts and each part is at the disposal of the whole. In the system is a kind of pseudohierarchy in the sense that our evolution is toward abstract thought, but this abstract thought rests on, is grounded in, is energized by, and is fed with associational data that enrich it so that it can grow. Within the 7 doorways model we refine not only the general principles of learning imprinted within students but also specific processes that we must use if, as Leslie Hart (1983) states, our schools are to be "brain compatible."

## Our Divided Oneness

All cultures have stories, myths, psychologies, philosophies, and spiritualities that describe human beings as fundamentally divided. We even hyperbolize this division when we say that one hand doesn't know what the other is doing. Neuroscientific research has revealed that our brains are the orchestrating mechanisms of this division. Certain functions are more or less localized, yet they share in a whole-brain grid of operations that helps each location become more perfect in its function. There are times, however, when one location seems not to know what another is doing. For educators, such neuroscientific information suggests a blueprint, an innate model for teaching and learning based on the organization and structure of the brain.

The way in which we see is one example of such duality. Objects presented to the left visual field of each eye are organized in the visual cortex of the right hemisphere. The visual cortex in the left hemisphere organizes data presented to the right visual field of each eye.

Communication between the hemispheres is radically decreased when the bundle of nerve fibers called the *corpus callosum,* which connects the left and right hemispheres, is severed. It becomes almost literally true that what one hemisphere is processing visually cannot be substantially communicated to the other hemisphere. Such communication failure leads to interesting responses to external stimuli.

Using vision to illustrate the dual processes of the brain, Michael Gazzaniga (1988) describes an experiment using subjects who have had their corpus callosum severed. He designed one test to evaluate their responses to different external stimuli. A chicken claw was flashed to participants' right visual field (the left hemisphere), while a snow scene was flashed to the left visual field (the right hemisphere). Participants were then shown a series of pictures and asked to pick two pictures associated with the chicken claw and the snow scene. The right hand, controlled by the left hemisphere, pointed to a chicken. The left hand, controlled by the right hemisphere, pointed to a shovel. The left hemisphere, which is the verbal hemisphere for 90 to 95 percent of the population, explained that the left hand chose the shovel because a shovel is used to clean out a chicken shed. Not knowing what the right hemisphere saw, the verbal hemisphere orchestrated a logical reason for what the left hemisphere saw.

Why is this experiment so important for teachers? It demonstrates the left hemisphere's blueprint for logical and interpretive verbal activity. It also points out the distance between logic and reality in certain situations. Sometimes even the smartest people with fully intact brains exhibit a shutdown between hemispheres—times when the verbal hemisphere attempts to rationalize what is more heavily impacting the right hemisphere. Learned behavior (repression) and schooling (control) require at least the pretense of this shutdown. We are a culture in conflict; we habitually censor perceptions, actions, and energy that flow in nonverbal ways through our bodies and minds.

At the elementary level the conflict between whole language and phonics dramatizes the rationalization and censoring tendencies in our thought processes. Although phonics has a place in teaching reading, using phonics alone can blind one to the successes of the whole-language methodology. Given the spatial functions of the right hemisphere coupled with interesting literature, a child may become a voracious reader who uses context clues to decode a book. Teachers may resist or cancel whole-brain approaches, however, when parents get jittery because their children are not skillful in recognizing individual words, even if the children are reading with overall comprehension and enjoyment. The verbal and logical left hemisphere debunks the whole-language approach by devising an explanation that ignores development in reading comprehension guided by right-hemisphere spatial and contextual skills. Wouldn't it be more logical to use whatever works for individual students?

Some of the most dramatic developmental changes occur in the bodies and minds of students at the middle-school level. These students are sexual, intuitive, experimental, independent, and are pulled both by childhood memories and adult fantasies; they ache for acceptance as well as for outlets for their diverse and sometimes cacophonous energies. The greatest harm that schools can do during these years is to frame an educational program in too sequenced and abstract a manner. One reason so many teachers burn out at the seventh-grade level is they try to censor and control right-brain tendencies and focus on left-brain activities, while this epoch in a child's growth and development requires teachers who are not censoring, who do not try to put a verbal/logical stranglehold on what is largely a right-brain phenomenon.

At the secondary level the gravest mistake teachers make is to assume that only students who are able to express themselves with highly organized and logically sequenced words are advancing their formal and abstract reasoning skills. In fact, we often use only verbal approaches to teach abstract reasoning skills. We ignore the role that visual, auditory, and kinesthetic experiences should play in the development of abstract reasoning because our narrow viewpoint blesses the construction of thought only when it is expressed in logical, verbal terms. We view the saying "a picture is worth a thousand words" as naive. An old-world, male-dominated censoring of abstraction is an entrenched framework for too much that goes on at the secondary level. A logic of fear must give way to the spectrum of expression so that the left hemisphere is not com-pelled to explain away what it would do best to understand in the first place.

## Cover-up: An Activity Where Left Meets Right

The purpose of this activity is to enable you to experience our tendency to cover up nonverbal experience. You will sense how this tendency often causes resistance to and fear of change in educational institutions, and also causes teachers to water down curricula that may otherwise challenge and relax.

Videotape two teachers as they tell lies about themselves. Afterward, both teachers should view the tape and take notes about how they felt while they were lying as well as what vocal and physical cues they think they gave. Show the tapes to a group of teachers and ask them to jot down notes about any nonverbal cues they notice in the speakers that might give away the fact that the speakers are lying. Afterward, brainstorm a list of cues that the group has observed and discuss why, even though these cues occur, we often disregard them. Next, to help participants ground this experience using both verbal and visual expression, have them write a piece of poetry or an expository essay grappling with the often censoring role the verbal hemisphere plays when faced with uncomfortable or perplexing nonverbal information. Have them give their pieces appropriate titles.

Next have the group study the two brush-stroke portraits of faces (see figure 1). Make two lists for each (a total of four lists), one that attempts to be as logical and analytical as possible and one that tries to let go and "feel into" each portrait. The participants will compare their own responses and then compare their responses with those of others in the group.

One analytical/logical comment about the first portrait might be that the paucity of lines allows the viewer to read into it anything he or she wants. Based on such a comment, a participant may conclude that we cannot reach an objective agreement about the meaning of art. Such a conclusion is logical and probably of some merit, but it says nothing about how the viewer actually "sees" the painting. A second response that is both logical and receptive to nonverbal information (feeling, spatial and symbolic themes) might be that the face at first appears stern, maybe sad, but on further study it appears to have a comical, almost lighthearted, nuance, perhaps expressing wisdom.

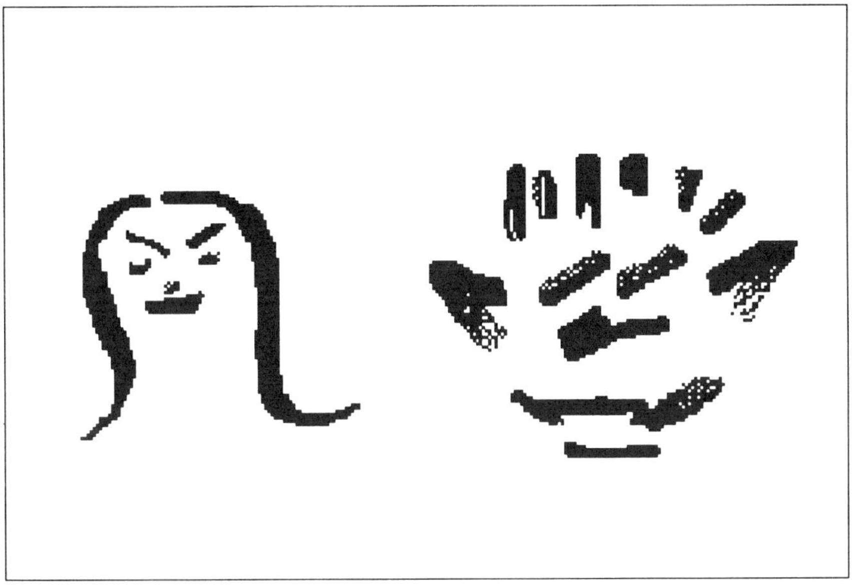

Figure 1. Two brush-stroke portraits of faces

An analytical/logical reaction to the second portrait might be that the minimalist approach could be the artist's attempt to equate simplicity with genius after the manner and style of a Picasso, but the net effect is no better than the uncultivated and uninspiring footprint of a family dog that entered the house through a mud puddle. Again, this comment seems perceptive and, perhaps, accurately critical of the artistic merit presented. On the other hand it serves to hide the personal dimension of the writer's experience of the art, which may have triggered some association with a person, an idea, or an autobiographical memory.

Jane M. Healy (1990) stresses the importance of coordinating the potentials of the fundamental duality at the heart of whole-brain learning:

> As both hemispheres work in tandem, they constantly toss the mental ball back and forth as they deal with different aspects of a problem. Some educators have suggested that children of today are more "right brained" because they rely too heavily on abilities commonly associated with the right hemisphere to handle academic "balls" that should be fielded by the left. It is true that traditional school-oriented tasks such as reading, spelling, computing accurately, writing

> logically, and reasoning analytically depend heavily on left hemisphere systems, but they cannot be accomplished without the help of the right. The critical question, therefore, is really not if children are "right brained" but if their environments are equipping them to use both hemispheres interactively. (128)

We must shift to learning models that truly integrate learning and accept the duality of human nature if we are to commit to a fundamental change in the way we run our schools. We cannot reverse gears once we have made the choice. We must struggle to go forward or suffer greater pain as a society and risk greater knee-jerk centralized control over our lives.

While children are being squeezed and shaped during their formative years into thoughtless, stimulus-response–driven consumers and their imaginations are being dried up by schools in financial or psychological turmoil, they feel most threatened by the possibility of abandonment. Like it or not, teachers are significant adult others in the lives of children. Sometimes a teacher is the only significant adult other. Youngsters often arrive at our schools emotionally torn, isolated from a sense of family, and adrift in a sea of meaningless confusion and apathy. Such feelings occur across the socioeconomic spectrum, from inner-city to bedroom-community school systems. The learning process must deal with this reality, and to do so teachers must capitalize on the real experience of kids as it flows through nonverbal messages in search of the verbal and the visual, which will give it a voice, the structure it seeks, and the dialogue of insight and understanding it requires.

It is in our power to make contact, to move into the circle of students' perceptions, conceptions, and feelings in order to help them help themselves. We are not substitute psychiatrists, pseudo–social workers, or mavens of moral righteousness. We are teachers: purveyors and surveyors of the power of knowledge; detectors and selectors of ability, talent, and motivation; callers to curiosity; touchstones for tomorrow's civilized world; and the bridge between hemispheres, a second corpus callosum, organizing the interface between the two basic selves that march through our schools and whom we call students.

In the final analysis we are many children's or teenagers' last opportunity to become excited about life. For the lucky children who come nurtured to our classrooms, we are the chance of a lifetime to expand their horizons, to build on their dreams, and to break through the narcissism of the family gradually in order to become both knowledgeable and compassionate human beings. Only teachers who are shifting and facing life as a whole themselves can offer that same experience to children. For those who have made the choice it is both a trying and enormously satisfying letting go of control. It is for those teachers who have already let go or who are looking for that one special something to begin the shift that the 7 Doorways model is intended.

# 1. THE 7 DOORWAYS MODEL
## A Glimpse

*Of Magic Doors*
*there is this:*
*you do not see them*
*even as you are*
*passing through.*

—John Pearson, *Magic Doors*

The duality I have described has been observable in humanity since the dawn of awareness. In recent years the neurosciences have contributed to our understanding of that duality, providing the basis for an absolute model of human learning that transcends culture and circumstance.

Although the 7 Doorways model has its conceptual basis in the neurosciences, one need not be aware of neuroscientific research to understand the model; we can observe in people's behavior the processes with which the model deals. Whether or not neuroscientists shift their understanding of the neural locus of brain functions, the 7 Doorways model will remain legitimate. The doorways describe thematic ways we learn, and both brain function and observable behavior legitimize the doorways.

Many teachers pass through these doorways daily. Others have tended to open and close just a few doors in their pattern of teaching. But the model is a natural process; teachers find themselves on the other side doing what they do best. What the 7 Doorways model offers is the opportunity to plan according to a model that arises from an "inner blueprint" and centuries of observation of human behavior.

## Doorway 1

Doorway 1 leads to a large neural area popularly referred to as the "left brain." The left brain processes information that is time bound, analytical, and fragmented, and that requires a syntactical, logical flow of words. Systems of written, oral, and auditory language are grounded here. The left brain structures reality into sequential bits and step-by-step arrangements according to a sense of time, causal chains of "before" and "after." The sign that hangs from Doorway 1 is *causation.*

## Doorway 2

Doorway 2 leads to a large neural area popularly referred to as the "right brain." The right brain processes images, spatial relationships, synthetic and holistic perceptions, and nonlinear, time-free information. It has rich connections with both affective and memory systems in the limbic areas. Because it processes globally, it may derive results and solutions to problems without laboring systematically through a series of carefully designed logical steps. Sometimes it seems to pluck data out of nowhere as do "autistic savants." It acts with a psychological radar, detecting all manner and species of nonverbal cues in the communication process. And, again because of its global motif, it makes associations that are the basis of rich metaphor. The sign that hangs from Doorway 2 is *intuition.*

## Doorway 3

Doorway 3 leads to a neural awareness network that controls brain-body, systemwide alertness. This network filters out and selects the information coming into Doorways 1 and 2 that requires immediate attention and processing. Without this "waiting room" function there would be too much data for the brain to deal with, and the whole system would lose its focus (as is the case with people who have attention-deficit disorders).

This doorway modulates attention between two polarities: rest and agitation. Its gatekeeper function legitimizes information that is new and unusual. It also acts as a kind of sixth-sense detector of the vibrations in the environment and tends to process ritual and familiar behavior as well as imitative, mimetic activity. It houses long-term physical memory, such as bike riding, and participates in homeostatic functions such as pulse, heart beat, blinking, and anything else that takes place automatically beneath consciousness. The sign that hangs from Doorway 3 is *automation.*

## Doorway 4

Doorway 4 opens to a neural forest in the right limbic region filled with all manner of emotional life and the affective elements in human communication. This region codes all learning with affective labels of like or dislike, love or hate. The region's primary focus is on self and others. The value it places on self and others colors our disposition to learn. Children who have low self-esteem or who dislike their teachers learn little. The teacher must resolve any conflicts before children can learn.

Doorway 4 participates in the gatekeeping function begun by Doorway 3. Doorway 3 will not admit for higher cortical examination any information Doorway 4 codes negatively unless Doorway 3 is highly motivated in other ways to do so. Energy becomes intensified in the limbic region, resulting in the well-known "fight or flight" response. Because this area is at the crossroads of neural circuitry, it contributes to associational memory and associational learning. The sign that hangs from Doorway 4 is *relation.*

## Doorway 5

Doorway 5 opens to neural operations that occur in the uppermost left limbic area of the brain. These operations are kin to those of Doorway 1 and govern maintenance of an orderly environment, ranging from the neatness of a desk or a room to the balancing and harmonizing of the demands of one's personal or professional life. We might easily label

Doorway 5 the clerical doorway, but for our purposes the sign that hangs from Doorway 5 is *administration.*

## Doorway 6

Doorway 6 leads to the area located above the eyebrows that sits on top and in front of the cerebral cortex. This area was the latest to develop in our evolution and it straddles both hemispheres. It comprises the frontal and prefrontal cortex. Neuroscientists now believe that this area of the brain determines our purpose and goals in life and serves as the repository of neural activity that channels the drive, will, and motivational energy necessary for the accomplishment of immediate and long-range goals.

This doorway is sometimes referred to as the executive branch of the brain. With information from both sides of the brain, this area gets a view of both the verbal and nonverbal data necessary to make informed decisions. An important element in decision making is the ability to look ahead and to forecast outcomes. The sign that hangs from Doorway 6 is *motivation.*

## Doorway 7

Doorway 7 leads to a region that spans the top of the neocortex from one ear to the other, the *sensorimotor cortex*. This region controls small- and large-muscle movement throughout the body. Early in life, females are generally small muscle oriented and males, large muscle oriented. Because we have misread this inner blueprint, we often expect young boys to become more language perfect than they can become, which results in a disproportionate number of boys in special education. The sign that hangs from this doorway is *motion.*

## The Complete Model

The 7 Doorways model encompasses models of left and right as well as up and down and contains within it the seeds of other learning models and personality types (see figure 1.1). This holistic model is based on seven fundamental functions of the brain, observable not only via the neurosciences but also through empirically verifiable behavior patterns that appear to be innate. All the functions are interdependent. You can

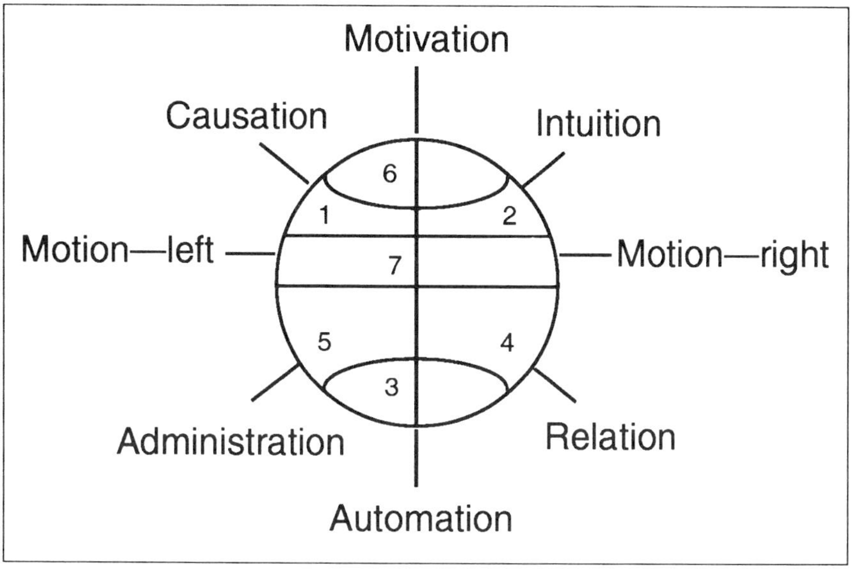


Figure 1.1. The complete 7 Doorways model

visualize this interdependence by imagining a large house with seven rooms. When you turn the light switch on in one room, it turns on the lights in the other rooms. Only the brightness and intensity of the lights differentiate one room from another.

This system is integrated. While tasks require neural action across the whole brain, the intensity of neural activity at any one location may be greater depending on genetics, culture, and schooling. The entire system depends on each of its parts and vice versa.

The model also has a two-directional masculine/feminine polarity. It possesses both the left/right and the up/down polarities of masculine/feminine. The left/right polarity contrasts causation with intuition while the up/down polarity contrasts motivation with automation. In general, the masculine half of the polarity is abstract and ungrounded, and the feminine half is embodied and grounded. A balance of these two halves makes the whole. Overemphasis on the masculine, or pure thought and order, results ironically in chaos and suppression. Overemphasis on the feminine creates stagnation and depression. The art and the science of whole-brain learning are in the play, sometimes uneven, between these extremes.

## The Embellished 7 Doorways Model

Imagine a grid overlapping the 7 Doorways model (see figure 1.2). Grid lines crisscross millions and millions of times in an infinitesimally fine thread, weaving a complicated interconnection. This enormously thick neural jungle of axons and dendrites is where the whole becomes sensitive to the parts and the parts to the whole. Paradoxically, any particular learning style is independent only insofar as it is dependent on all other learning styles. The 7 Doorways model supports a learning style theory that respects individual styles while calling for that style to stretch itself intentionally into the other domains.

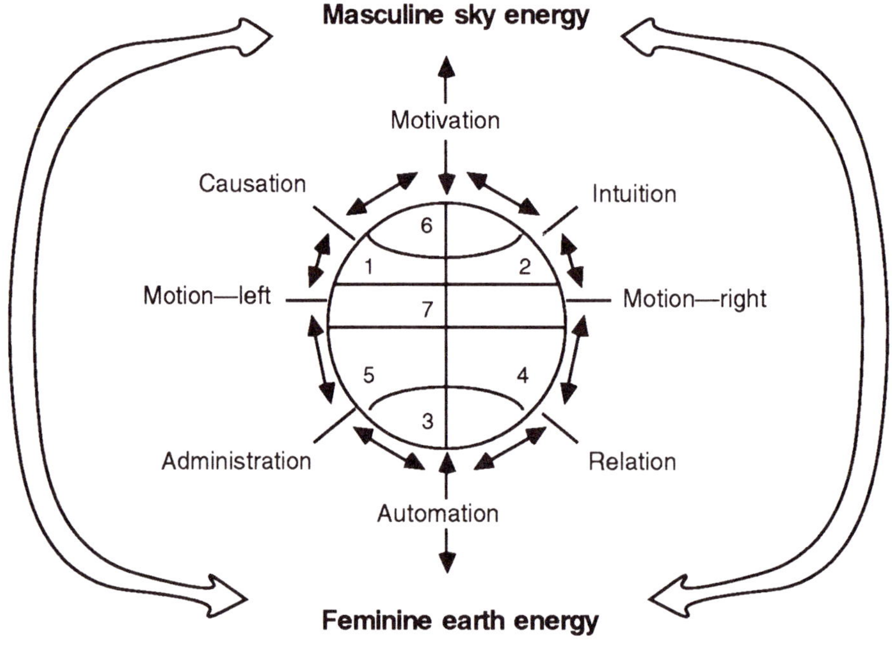


Figure 1.2. The embellished 7 Doorways model, showing the interconnections among the areas of the brain

## Teacher Perceptions Questionnaire

Read the following questions carefully. Answer them with either a yes or a no. Please don't answer with both. When you have finished answering the questions, quietly thumb through your daily newspaper, keeping track of articles that give you an idea of how our society is doing in terms of the 7 Doorways model. For example, an article on child abuse would reflect a negative experience inside Doorway 4, where relationships are important.

When you have finished scanning the newspaper, fill out the questionnaire again. Did your answers change? Have you gained a deeper sense of the social experiences that form and influence the 7 Doorways framework in the lives of your students?

## The Questionnaire

### Question

| *Doorway 1: Causation* | **Response 1** (Circle One) | **Response 2** (Circle One) |
|---|---|---|
| 1. Are today's children smarter than children in the past? | Yes No | Yes No |
| 2. Do today's children write better than children in the past? | Yes No | Yes No |
| 3. Do today's children think as logically as children did years ago? | Yes No | Yes No |
| 4. Do today's children express themselves orally as well as children did in the past? | Yes No | Yes No |
| ***Doorway 2: Intuition*** | | |
| 5. Are today's children more visual than children were in the past? | Yes No | Yes No |
| 6. Do today's children seem to have a better sixth sense than children did years ago? | Yes No | Yes No |
| 7. Do you find that today's children seem to understand something but can't immediately explain it more frequently than children in the past? | Yes No | Yes No |

8. Do today's children write better poetry than children did in years gone by? Yes No Yes No

*Doorway 3: Automation*

9. Do today's children seem more relaxed and less stressed than children in the past? Yes No Yes No

10. Do today's children seem to be involved more with nature than children were in the past? Yes No Yes No

11. Do today's children seem as bonded to significant adults as children were in the past? Yes No Yes No

12. Do today's rituals of play seem as good today as they were in the past? Yes No Yes No

***Doorway 4: Relation***

13. Do today's children seem to have lower self-esteem than children used to? Yes No Yes No

14. Are today's children more abused and neglected than children used to be? Yes No Yes No

15. Are today's children more violent than children in the past? Yes No Yes No

16. Are today's children more concerned for others than children were years ago? Yes No Yes No

***Doorway 5: Administration***

17. Are today's children neater in their physical habits than children were in the past? Yes No Yes No

18. Can today's children organize themselves better than children could in the past? Yes No Yes No

| | | | | |
|---|---|---|---|---|
| 19. Can today's children balance the demands made on them today better than children could years ago? | Yes | No | Yes | No |
| 20. Are the study habits of today's children better than those of children in the past? | Yes | No | Yes | No |

***Doorway 6: Motivation***

| | | | | |
|---|---|---|---|---|
| 21. Are today's children as motivated to learn as children were in years past? | Yes | No | Yes | No |
| 22. Are today's children as willful as children were in the past? | Yes | No | Yes | No |
| 23. Are today's children as goal oriented as children were in the past? | Yes | No | Yes | No |
| 24. Do today's children have as much a sense of their own future as children did in the past? | Yes | No | Yes | No |

***Doorway 7: Motion***

| | | | | |
|---|---|---|---|---|
| 25. Do today's children have more problems staying still than children used to? | Yes | No | Yes | No |
| 26. Are today's children more athletic than children were in the past? | Yes | No | Yes | No |
| 27. Does it seem that today's children have more sensorimotor problems than children in the past? | Yes | No | Yes | No |
| 28. Have you observed a difference in the way today's children walk and hold their bodies compared to the way children held themselves in the past? | Yes | No | Yes | No |

When you have finished this exercise, you will have a cursory analysis of where you think children stand in relation to the 7 Doorways model. The next step is to answer the following question: *What can you do with this information to change what you do in the classroom?*

## Introductory Activities

The 7 Doorways model is the basis for the following sample lesson. You can implement the model in any K–12 classroom and in practically any discipline. Over time most teachers can get a real feel for the dynamic, open-ended, and natural qualities of the 7 Doorways model. You can use the model, among other things, as a tool for evaluating who your students are, what you might do with them, what you want to do with them, and what you are actually doing with them. Although familiarity with the model requires years of conscious and unconscious observing, planning, and experimenting, you need not wait that long to begin using it. You will have to do some preparation, such as creating a guided imagery for your students.

### Sample Lesson

Read the following story (or a story that is more relevant to your purposes):

The Chicken Crosses the Street

> Once upon a time there was a chicken who loved hamburgers. One day, the chicken spotted a restaurant that served what he heard were the best hamburgers in town. Because the chicken was afraid to enter the restaurant for fear he'd soon become food for the customers, he disguised himself as a young boy. He crossed the street and walked into the restaurant. He sat down at a table hoping that the cook wouldn't think he was a chicken just because he had a beak. A tall man dressed as a waiter walked over to the chicken.

Read the following activities and add to them so that you end up with a series of choices in each category.

*Doorway 1: Causation*

- Have your students complete the story and explain why they chose the sequence of events.
- Have students create a list of questions about the story. Remind them to use "Why" and "What if" as starter words for a number of questions.
- Have students research whether or not a chicken would eat a hamburger and explain why it would or would not.
- Have students use a problem-solving format to figure out another way the chicken could get to eat a hamburger at the restaurant.

*Doorway 2: Intuition*

- Have students draw a chicken dressed up as a boy and label aspects of its attire so it looks like a poster they might see in a store.
- Have students create a story about the further adventures of the chicken. They will tape-record their stories with their eyes closed.
- Write a guided imagery that stresses as much sensory information as possible about the chicken's attempt to get served a hamburger. Play baroque music in the background and have your students relax. Read the guided imagery to your students and as soon as you are finished, have them write as much as they can about what they felt, saw, and experienced. Tell them they can go back later to proofread. They will also share the writing with the class.
- Have students write a poem in which they make several comparisons about the chicken.

*Doorway 3: Automation*

- Have students imitate a chicken while they try to walk along a straight line you draw in chalk on the floor.
- Have students create a chicken clan with chicken clan rituals that would precede a hunt for hamburgers.
- Have students mime the chicken in the chicken story.
- Divide students into groups of ten or more. They will pretend they are chickens sitting as quietly as they can in the chicken coop. Remind them to pay attention to how they feel, restful or anxious. They will share their feelings with classmates.

*Doorway 4: Relation*

- Have students interview the chicken. They will ask him questions such as, "What is it like being a chicken in a world where you have to wear a disguise?"
- Have students write a poem, an essay, or a story about what it's like to grow up as a chicken.
- Have students role-play the customer relations department in a store. The department must deal with complaints from chickens about items the store sells only to the chickens.
- Have students create a chicken advice column (Ann Landers style) in which students give advice to chickens with problems.

*Doorway 5: Administration*

Divide students into groups or "chicken coops." They will assign roles to each member of the coop and agree on a list of rules that meet the needs of each chicken.

- Have students write a series of five memos to the chicken coops that tell the coops what they need to do to keep up egg production, sales, and profits.
- Have students call a meeting of representatives from each coop, hand out a written agenda for the meeting, and run the meeting. They will send minutes of the meeting to each representative.
- Have students create a questionnaire that assesses how well organized and happy each coop is. Publish the results and list ideas to deal with any problems.

*Doorway 6: Motivation*

- Have students develop a contest with real prizes for the best individual and team ideas for how the chicken can get what he wants—hamburgers.
- Have students form forecasting groups. Have each group create lists of forecasts concerning what will happen to the chicken industry in a hundred years. Let the groups compare, discuss, and negotiate a final large-group forecast.
- Divide the class into two groups, the causation group and the intuition group. The causation group gathers verbal information

about chickens. The intuition group gathers nonverbal information (pictures, images, music, and so on) about chicken life. The groups pool their information in order to decide the answer to the following question: Will chickens look different in the year 2000? After each group answers this question, have the whole group decide what kind of information is missing that would enable them to answer the question more realistically.

- Using the same groups as in the previous exercise, have them answer the question, "Do chickens want to be chickens?" The causation group will speak as logically and precisely as possible, and the intuition group will use imagination, spontaneous art, charts and diagrams, even dramatic renditions or on-the-spot video. Afterward have each group comment on how they benefitted from the presentation of the other group.

*Doorway 7: Motion*

- Have students form a line. Toss a sponge football to each student in turn. The first child who catches the ball must ask a question about chickens. The next child to catch the ball must answer the question. Continue the game until each student has asked and answered a question.
- Play "Simon Says"; at some point say, "Simon says, 'Raise your hand if you want to answer a question.'" Place those who raise their hands in a group. Then say to this group, "Simon says, 'Step forward if you want to answer a difficult question.'" Continue narrowing the group in this way until you have one person left. That person will pick five other students and they will write questions about chickens. They will ask the class the questions and get a prize for every question that stumps the class.
- Divide the students into pairs. The pairs will take turns. When it is a pair's turn, the class tosses out a topic that concerns chickens. The pair walks around the classroom discussing the topic. Strongly suggest the pairs ask each other questions in their conversation.
- Have the students count off in sixes. The ones will comprise a team, the twos will comprise a team, and so on. Then divide the students into groups of six each, with one member from each team in each

group. Each group of six will lie on the floor in a circle with their feet pointed toward the middle of the circle. Decide what movement students will make if they know the answer to a question. A student may raise a hand, raise both hands, do a sit up, and so forth. Ask each group of six a question about chickens. Teams score one point if their member of the group is the first to make the appropriate movement, be recognized, and answer the question correctly. When you have asked the first group a question and someone has answered it correctly, ask the next group a question. Continue the game until one team gets six points.

### What the Activities Suggest

The activities suggest that you can address any content through the 7 Doorways model. The activities also suggest that it is easier than you might have thought to create interdisciplinary approaches to subject matter. You will see how to apply the 7 Doorways model to different subject matter in later chapters, especially if you are willing to put in the time to create activities focused on content across the disciplines, to have kids select the activities, to enable the kids to organize themselves, and to balance teaching in front of the class with a roaming, facilitating teaching style.

Using the 7 Doorways model will change the structure of your class gradually so that students interact, discuss, and create more. The model will also make your content relevant and bring it alive, even in areas that are usually difficult for students, such as literary classics. Each class, however, requires you to judge how much you need to control the content, process, and product rather than facilitating them. In classes where attendance patterns are erratic, you may need to control the content more, incorporating your activities based on the 7 Doorways model. You will need to design the activities for large groups, except in instances where you can create a challenging game.

## Conclusion

Figure 1.3 provides you with an overview of chapter 1. You may copy it to use as a handy reference for the activities and attitudes that each doorway comprises.

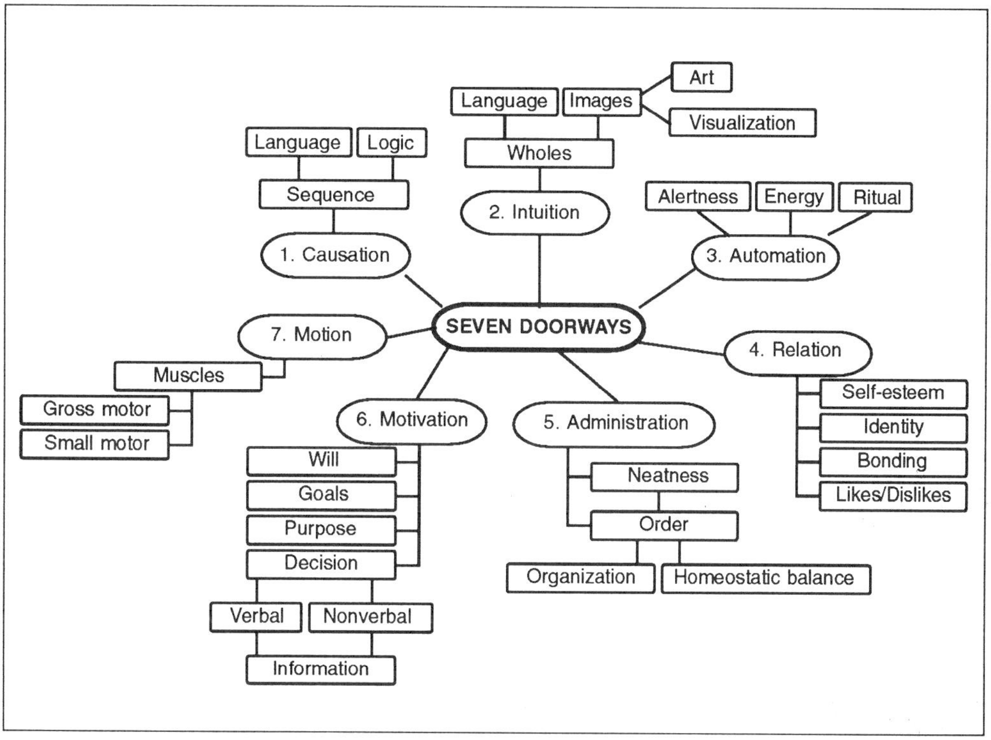


Figure 1.3. Webbed summary of chapter 1

# 2. CAUSATION

> *It is possible to teach thinking skills, and it is essential for people who will be faced with choices and decisions all their lives to develop these skills as early as possible.*
>
> —Herbert Kohl, *Basic Skills*

Doorway 1, causation, can be likened to what is stereotypically referred to as "the left brain." It deals primarily with *causal chains of information.* Causal chains of information are *sequenced bits and pieces of data* that flow from each other in a time-bound package.

## Language

The primary causal information chain is language itself. The grammar and syntax of a language are inherently logical, and we learn these patterns at an early age. For example, a child learns to say "I want my mommy" rather than "Want mommy my I." One word follows another to form a comprehensible statement. The chain of words is causally linked in a sequence that is time bound: one word precedes the next word, which precedes the next word, which together cause meaning.

## Causality Defined

Peter A. Angeles (1981) defines *cause* as "anything capable of changing something else" and "that which 'produces' something ('makes' something happen; 'brings about' the occurrence of something) without which that thing would not have resulted. That which is produced (or changed) is called the effect and the effect is explained by its cause" (s.v. "cause").

The idea that causation is a *bringing about* process is fundamental to all thought. Babies are always looking for results, and although this search takes place in the trancelike state of infancy, it is nevertheless a causal process. When the baby moves to the mother's breast and is satisfied by feeding, the baby is taking part in the causal process, and the brain is developing its "if this, then that" connectivity.

What differentiates infancy, childhood, adolescence, and adulthood in the causation process is the scope of conscious awareness of and the verbal ability to deal with the process. Someday the toddler will think, "If I pick up my toys, I can have a piece of gum." An adolescent may say, "If I do well on my report card, I can use the car." Someday an adult might consider, "If I get what I want, will happiness follow?"

## Consequences

We can look at causation from the perspective of consequences. Consequences become verbalized more precisely as the process of logical thought develops. As with everything in life, the richer the field of experiences, the more sophisticated will be one's understanding of consequences. Limited life experiences create limited awareness of consequences and limited ability to verbalize the relationships between things. Essential to the development of the awareness of consequences and verbal processing of the relationships between events is the *freedom to ask questions*. Rather than always giving answers, teachers can help students immensely by encouraging students to ask questions across the curriculum.

## The Four Causes

Aristotle (384–322 B.C.E.) wrote of four basic causes by which the existence of anything can be understood. We can ask questions that help students understand the four different causes. When we ask the question "What is this made of?" we are looking for the *material cause*. When we ask "What is this thing?" or "What is it meant to be?" we are looking for the *formal cause*. When we ask "Who or what made this?" we are looking for the *efficient cause*. When we ask "What is the purpose or goal for this thing?" we are looking for the *final cause*.

Teaching always implicitly involves the four causes. For example, if we are discussing the Atlantic Ocean we might set up our lesson plan as follows:

1. What is the ocean made of? (material cause)
2. What makes an ocean an ocean and not a river? (formal cause)
3. What formed the oceans and how did they come about? (efficient cause)
4. Why do oceans exist? (final cause)

Such questions help students develop skills in causal analysis, which is a property of Doorway 1.

## Individuals and Classes

Although only individual objects seem to exist, they share enough qualities to form a class. Children might experience the texture, solidity, and feel of hard objects, for example. Over time the repeated experience of these qualities would enable children to see similarities in hard objects and to classify them as such. This process of classification is dependent on causal and consequential thinking.

The art of classification is governed by logical laws. Bertrand Russell (1960) reminds us that what is true of one thing is not necessarily true of the class to which it belongs. He says,

> If in any sentence in which a thing is mentioned, you substitute a class for a thing, you no longer have a sentence that has any meaning: the sentence is no longer either true or false but a meaningless collection of words. For example, in the sentence, 'Adam is fond of apples,' you may substitute mankind, and say, 'Mankind is fond of apples.' But obviously you do not mean there is one individual, called 'Mankind,' which munches apples; you mean that the separate individuals who compose mankind are each severally fond of apples. (160)

When we determine classes, we must be careful not to assume that people fit wholly or irrevocably into a given class. For example, an individual who is fat may belong to a class called obese people, but if the individual loses weight, he or she no longer belongs to that class. Classifying people, places, or objects requires analyzing what they share and being careful not to generalize about individuals within the class or to categorize without sufficient evidence. If two people share one characteristic, they do not necessarily share a third, or if one person who belongs to a class of people is a bigot, the class to which she belongs is not thereby bigoted. The mistake of judging a whole group of people based on the actions of one is at the heart of all sorts of prejudice.

You can challenge young children enormously by asking them to find qualities that objects, places, and persons share and to classify the items accordingly. You can present older children and teenagers with classifications and ask the students to evaluate the quality of the classifications. Classifying is fundamental to writing essays and reports, as well as to discussing human problems such as racism and drug abuse.

Some of the difficulties students and teachers have with each other flow from classification errors. Students might classify a teacher as "strict" or "judgmental" and assume all teachers are strict and judgmental. Or teachers might classify students as "poor readers" or "discipline problems," seeing the students only in the light of how well they do certain tasks.

## Logic

*Deductive logic* requires using a principle or a classification and drawing a conclusion about individuals based on it. The classical expression of deductive logic is propositional logic:

All men are thinkers.
Harry is a man.
Therefore, Harry is a thinker.

The flow of thought is from the general to the particular. At any step along the way, however, one can make an error. If the generalization is untrue, then what follows is not necessarily true. If the middle is false, then one cannot conclude what follows.

*Inductive logic* requires the development of a generalization from a series of particulars that together suggest a classification. Scientists create and test their theories by reasoning inductively. If you see enough sunrises in a succession of days, you might inductively arrive at the theory that the sun will always rise once in every twenty-four-hour period.

Do students exercise these logical formats? Most of the time. Are the conclusions students arrive at always valid? No. The teacher must check the premises by which students draw conclusions as well as the data from which they induct a principle or a theory. If teachers can help students to check logic for themselves, teachers will have taught the students a great deal.

## Analysis

Analysis is derived from a Greek term meaning "to unloose." Doorway 1 concerns itself with taking wholes and "unloosing" their constituent parts in order to study the parts and how they contribute to the whole. Many teachers recognize this concept from Bloom's taxonomy. Children are always taking things apart and attempting to reconstruct them or to find alternative uses for them. Teachers can enhance students' development of analytical skills behind Doorway 1 by supplying children with manipulatives the children can pull apart ("unloosen") and put back together. The process will transfer into problem-solving skills whereby language, causality, classification, and logic become ever more conscious and controlled tools of thought.

## Key Words

Following is a list of key words representing concepts, processes, and seed ideas that I include here because they are Doorway 1 priorities:

analysis
argument (to make clear)
concept
connotation
conversation
denotation
ends
equivocation
evidence
explication
fact
fallacy
hypothesis
idea
implication
inference
inquiry
means
metaphor
opinion
paradox
philosophy
precept
principles
probability
questioning
scientific method
semantics
socratic method
syllogism
synthesis
system
themes
theory

What would you say if someone told you that children make great philosophers? Their natural curiosity, awe, wonder, and puzzlement are exhibited in their interesting questions and their conversations that only the most biased of adults would dismiss as meaningless. Gareth Mathews (1980) offers the following questions and comments:

- A six-year-old asked, "Papa, how can we be sure everything is not a dream?" (1).
- A five-year-old asked, "If I go to bed at eight and get up at seven in the morning, how do I really know that the little hand of the clock has gone around only once?" (2).
- An eight-year-old asked, "Daddy, why don't I see you double because I have two eyes and I can see you with each one by itself?" (8).
- A six-year-old stated, "Early and late aren't things. They're not things like tables and chairs and cups—things you can model." (14).
- A three-year-old responded to her mother's observation that the toddler's tummyache would go away if she were to lie down: "Where will it go?" (17).
- A six-year-old asked, "Which part of me is really me?" (86).

It appears that young children make statements of all kinds that are experimental, playful, and meaningful. Most developmental and cognitive scientists have focused only on the experimental and playful aspects of children's language and have denied there is any serious intentional, inquisitory meaning.

"On the contrary," states Mathews (1980). "In fact, such evidence as I have been able to assemble suggests that for many young members of the human race, philosophical thinking—including on occasion subtle and ingenious reasoning—is as natural as making music and playing games, and quite as much a part of being human" (36). Mathews quite rightly asserts that children's whimsical questions, responses to stories, and ability to sustain conversations demonstrate empirically that there is more going on in their linguistic expression than a simple romantic toying with words.

Lipman, Oscanyan, and Sharp (1984) include the following list of themes and ideas in a much larger list meant for discussion and writing in grades 4–7:

| | |
|---|---|
| inquiry | doubt |
| discovery and invention | trust |
| thinking | duty |
| logical statement | possibility |
| truth | art and life |
| good and right | innocence (iii–vii) |
| value | |

You might be amazed that children at these grade levels can deal with such abstraction. It is possible because the abstract ideas are grounded in the story so that the inquiry is not forced and does not violate the student's developmental readiness.

## Critical Skills

Eppig, Knowles, and Monether (1989) list the following skills as "vital to the success of any individual in today's complex and changing society" (12):

1. Problem solving
2. Decision making
3. Critical thinking
4. Creative thinking
5. Communication
6. Organization
7. Cooperation/Collaboration
8. Management
9. Leadership
10. Independent learning
11. Documentation

Numbers 1, 3, 5, 6, 8, 10, and 11 are skills that involve processes that exist behind Doorway 1. For example, *critical thinking* depends on analysis of data; *communication* requires accurate listening, clear speech, and precise writing; *organization* requires prioritizing and managing time and tasks; *management* requires a thorough understanding of organizational structure; *independent learning* requires problem-solving ability; and *documentation* involves keeping accurate, detailed notes. All these skills require students to use their brains in a special way in which causation and all processes related to causation are paramount.

## Values and Ethics

The last major subtopic that characterizes Doorway 1 comes from the moral and aesthetic realm. What is right? How do we know it is right? And why do people's beliefs about right and wrong differ? What is beauty? How do we know it is beauty? And why do people's beliefs about beauty differ?

Lawrence Kohlberg created neat, developmentally aligned categories that provide indicators of why people behave as they do. He defines the six main stages in the development of moral reasoning: (1) punishment and obedience compel moral behavior; (2) personal usefulness motivates moral decisions; (3) conforming to the will of the group is the basis for action; (4) law and order become ends in themselves and the foundation for behavior; (5) social contract, constitutionalism, and higher laws are a basis for behavior and the right to act; and (6) personal conscience guided by universal moral law honoring distributive justice, human rights, and the dignity of individuals forms the basis of moral action (Clark 1983, 112–15).

Doorway 1 is the arena that distinguishes means from ends and causes from effects in relation to right action. Children live amid a ceaseless flow of events that require the children to make decisions that are laden with consequences. Through the relationship between decision and consequence the child learns cause and effect. Because understanding consequences leads to appropriate behavior, and appropriate behavior in the classroom is necessary, Doorway 1 is probably the first area of rational concern between children and their teachers.

It is probably the category of beauty that truly evokes early preconscious and conscious forays for children, teens, and adults into the moral domain and, by intrinsic logic, into the causal domain. At first we distinguish between angels and monsters, then handsome and homely, and finally a healthy ecology and destruction. Beauty and ugliness, life and decay, draw the evolving consciousness into the causal connections between choice, action, and consequence. This arena is the playground of ecstasy and the scraped knee. It is where lessons are learned and moral reasoning developed.

## Doorway 1 Activities

You may adapt the following activities to use across the curriculum and across grade levels. The activities are based on the following story.

### The Chicken Who Wanted to Be an Eagle

> There was a chicken named Light-as-a-Feather who lived in a chicken coop made of petrified broccoli and old, stale potato chips. Sometimes when the chickens had little food they'd peck away at the coop. Over the years the coop got smaller and smaller—so small, in fact, that the coop was big enough for only one chicken, Light-as-a-Feather.
>
> The corn crop that summer was poor and by midwinter there was no food left for Light-as-a-Feather. Light-as-a-Feather had to make a decision. Should she begin to eat her home, to peck away at the broccoli and potato chips, and by doing so expose herself to the harsh

winter, or should she keep her warm coop and starve? Before she could make the decision, she ate the last bit of corn and left the coop to walk around in the midwinter sunshine to clear her head. In the sky, flying carelessly and smoothly about, was her eagle friend, Talon. Spotting Light-as-a-Feather below, Talon swooped down, and with great play in her heart, grabbed Light-as-a-Feather and lifted her high into the sky.

Light-as-a-Feather was afraid of flying and closed her eyes tightly. She was barely able to squeak out, "Wha . . . Wha . . . what's up? Where are you taking me, Talon?!" Talon felt Light-as-a-Feather jerk a little in her grasp, but her grip was firm and she flew on high to her aerie atop a tall tree that was firmly rooted in the side of a mountain overlooking a great river.

When they arrived at the nest, Talon let Light-as-a-Feather drop into it. The nest swayed a bit and settled as Talon circled to prepare for her landing next to Light-as-a-Feather.

Talon's claws reached out instinctively for the nest and Talon instantly crouched there as if she had never left in the first place. "What happened? Why'd you do this, Talon?" asked Light-as-a-Feather.

"Do what?" responded Talon.

"Oh, come, Talon, don't act dumb!" said Light-as-a-Feather. "I didn't get here on my own!"

"But you're here, and that's all that counts, so let's talk, Light, okay?" suggested Talon.

They talked for awhile until darkness covered the nest and the moon danced on the river. "I've got to go, Talon!" insisted Light-as-a-Feather "Take me home."

"Fly home yourself, Light, fly home yourself!" responded Talon.

Light-as-a-Feather looked Talon in the eye and yelled back, "I can't, I can't!"

There was silence. Talon nudged Light to the edge of the nest as if she were initiating an eagle chick into its first flight. "Move over, Talon! I'm gonna fall out!" erupted Light.

"No kidding, Light!" said Talon. With that Talon gave Light one final nudge out over the rim of the nest. Light's wings flapped madly as she fell like a rock through the cold night air. The air pressed like hands against her eyes, making them water and blurring her vision. Her feathers flew off her body like exploding white sparks, and the fear of hitting the ground like a raw hamburger made her shake so much that her wings flapped like high-speed fans and her fall was stopped in midair.

"I'm flying! Holy Gee! Heavens! I'm flying!" screamed Light-as-a-Feather.

"I knew you could," sounded Talon's familiar voice. With gently and rhythmically undulating wings, Talon had flown from the nest prepared to save Light if Light didn't learn the lesson. "Now, go home," said Talon, "go home."

When Light-as-a-Feather reached her broccoli-and-chips coop she had forgotten completely about her hunger. She slept well that night. When she awoke the next morning, her stomach growled. Her only thought was to find out from Talon how eagles find their food in the winter.

Following is a selection of Doorway 1 ideas for classroom activities. Although there are activities for each Doorway 1 subtopic, all the activities deal ultimately with causality, sequencing elements that logically precede and come after each other.

## Language Activities

- Create a list of questions about the story. Be sure some start with "why," "what if," and "should."
- Outline the story. Add at least five more events to the story and explain your placement of them.
- Role-play a press conference in which one student plays Light-as-a-Feather and the rest of the students play reporters asking questions. Allow as many students as possible to play Light or Talon during the "conference."
- Make a list of the best or most difficult words in the story and look up their definitions as well as synonyms.
- Continue the story by developing what happens after Light realizes she wants to find out how eagles hunt for food in winter.
- Re-create the story in another verbal medium, such as poetry or dramatic dialogue.
- List five things Light learns from her experience, then arrange them in the order of their importance. Explain why you put them in this order.
- Write the separate words from the opening of the story on pieces of large paper. Lay them face up on a table and mix them up. Divide students into teams and have them reconstruct the story by placing the words in the correct order.

- On small pieces of paper write individual words that describe the characters' positive and negative characteristics. Place the pieces of paper in a bowl. Have students come up to the bowl one at a time, pick a characteristic, and explain clearly how it applies or does not apply to either Light or Talon. Other students then ask the student questions.
- I suggest the following model, first paragraph design, as one way to teach students how to organize an essay. The model allows students to master organization of verbal expression across the disciplines, so it is useful in areas besides language arts and English classes.

  The key to this model is the first paragraph of a written work from which the remaining paragraphs flow. The first sentence introduces the topic. Sentences 2, 3, and 4 state an aspect about the topic. Paragraph 2 explains sentence 2 from Paragraph 1. Paragraph 3 explains sentence 3 from Paragraph 1. Paragraph 4 explains sentence 4 from Paragraph 1. The fifth paragraph simply summarizes, looks back on what was stated, and ends with a concluding remark. Figure 2.1 illustrates how the paragraph will look.

  This model helps children organize their essays logically and judge the importance of the available information. The model may inhibit creativity at first because it demands a discipline to the writing, but students can develop paragraphs 2, 3, and 4 internally with a great deal of originality and creative spark. Because many children simply don't organize their writing, this simple and straightforward model will free them to think of writing as less of a chore and more of something enjoyable, as it should be. Be sure, however, that your students know this is a beginning model and that most essays have more than three well-developed main ideas.

- Another way students can ensure their writing is organized is to have them develop an outline *after* they have written an essay. Since we often write to discover, insisting that students develop an outline before they write and stick to it does not work well. But if they outline their completed essays, students can see easily which ideas don't belong, which need more development, or which need to be moved. They can also determine whether each idea flows into

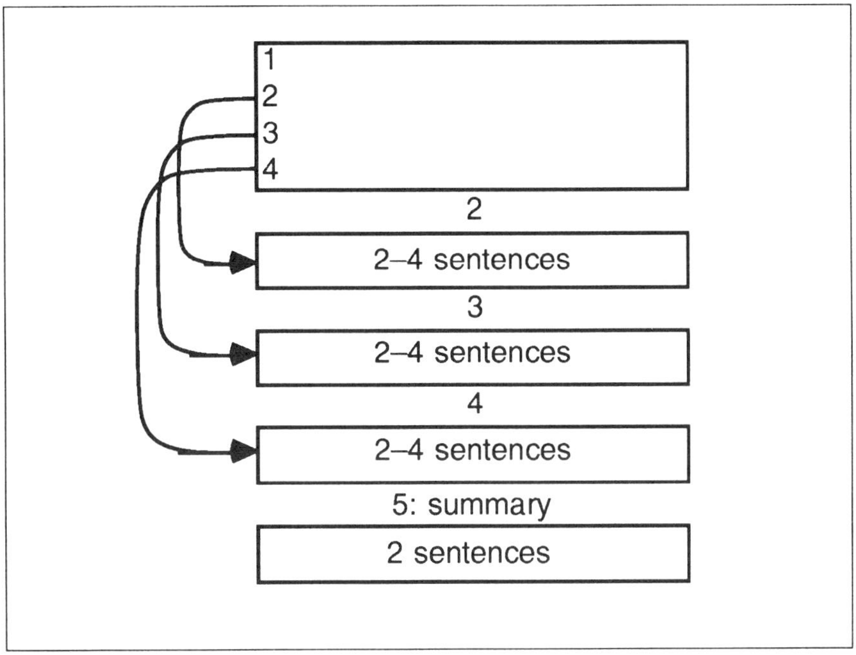


Figure 2.1. First paragraph design

the next logically. Students who don't have trouble getting a lot of ideas down on paper will find this technique useful.

## Causality Activities

- List all causes and effects that the story contains, then list them in the order of their importance.
- What other cause/effect relationships could have been included in the story? For example, had Light-as-a-Feather actually crashed and died, we would have to say that Talon caused her to die, that Talon killed Light-as-a-Feather.
- Create ten questions about the story that begin with "why." Answer each starting with "because."

## Four Causes Activity

For each of the four causes, create as many questions that apply to each of the items and characters in the chart that follows.

| | Final cause (Why was it made?) | Efficient cause (What made it?) | Formal cause (What was it meant to be?) | Material cause (What is it made of?) |
|---|---|---|---|---|
| Light-as-a-Feather | | | | |
| Talon | | | | |
| Light learning to fly | | | | |
| Talon's nest | | | | |

Based on your questions, write a report, essay, or dialogue using the four causes as the theme.

## Individual and Class Activities

- Using the parts of speech as categories, group the words from the first two paragraphs of the story.
- List the ways in which Light-as-a-Feather and Talon are physically and psychologically similar.
- Classify or give a tag name to the story. To what kind or group of stories does it belong?
- List animals that are in the same class as chickens and list those that are in the same class as eagles. Describe the characteristics that each class possesses and point out how the classes are different.

## Logic Exercises

- Based on the story, see if you can create a simple syllogism in which a third statement follows logically from the two that precede it. Here is a model:

  A. All human beings have parents. (universal)

  B. Shirley is a human being. (particular)

  C. Shirley has parents. (conclusion)

Be sure your syllogisms are like the model and that each element is in its correct place. Here is an example from the story:

A. All chickens have wings.

B. Light is a chicken.

C. Light has wings.

See how many syllogisms you can make based on the story and the characters.

- Using the story, write as many "If . . . , then . . . " statements as you can. Here is one example: *If Light wants to fly, then she will fly.* Is the statement logically correct?
- Create *analogies* (comparisons between two things that have something in common) about either Light-as-a-Feather or Talon. Here is an example from the story: *Light is like a book that has fallen from a shelf.* This statement refers to the moment when Light falls from Talon's nest. Although Light is not a book, she falls like a book, suddenly and quickly and heavily.
- Make as many "A-propositions" based on the story as you can. (An A-Proposition is a universal statement, such as "All chickens have wings.")
- Come up with as many noun ideas that represent the story as you can. Here are a few: success, fear, flight.
- A "condition" refers to circumstances that exist when something takes place. A "necessary condition" is a circumstance that is necessary for an event or action to take place. A "sufficient condition" is a circumstance under which the event always happens. Can you list conditions that exist in the story and explain why they are either "necessary" or "sufficient"? For example: *Light-as-a-Feather had to fall from Talon's nest in order to learn how to fly* (necessary condition).
- *A contradictory proposition* contains two statements, but only one statement is true, as in the following example:

All men have parents.

Some men have no parents.

If it is true that *all* men have parents it can never be true that *some* men have no parents. These propositions are therefore contradictory.

Write at least five sets of contradictory propositions based on the story. For example:

All chickens have wings.
Some chickens have no wings.

- In *contrary propositions,* both statements are false. Here's an example:

  All chickens speak Chinese.
  Only some chickens do not speak Chinese.

  Both of the propositions in this set are false. Write five sets of contrary propositions based on some elements from the story.
- The defining of terms is very important in formal arguments and when writing or speaking in order to prove or present a point of view. Define any term from the story, being sure that your definition contains one or more of the following: a synonym, examples, the classification to which the term belongs, and any differences it has from other members of that class.
- *Denotation* and *connotation* of words are also very important. *Denotation* is the ordinary definition of a word. *Connotation* is the extraordinary definition of a word influenced by culture and popular usage. Here is an example from the story:

  *Chicken:* two-legged feathered and flightless bird raised for food (denotation).

  *Chicken:* afraid or fearful of doing something (connotation).

  List at least ten words from the story and give denotative and connotative meanings for each.

## Analysis Activity

Make a list of the parts of a chicken and describe what they cost per pound to buy in a store. Create a step-by-step recipe for an original chicken dinner.

## Key-Word Activities

Have students find definitions for five of the key words, then have them develop an activity or demonstration for one of the terms.

## Philosophy Activities

- You can use any story as a basis for philosophical inquiry with kids. You can make the discussion easier by asking good questions, attempting to define terms, and listening attentively for possible directions suggested by children's responses.
- Give a group of children an array of objects and charge the children to play with the objects. Instruct the children to return to you periodically with a question about one or all of the objects. After you've collected the questions, gather the children in a circle and ask the whole group the questions.
- Assign students to write a dialogue about anything they choose; they must, however, explore the effect of the object, the experience, or the idea about which they choose to write. For example, have a team write a dialogue that explores the ultimate purpose of love.
- Place one object in the middle of the classroom. Before students touch or hold the object, have them list their observations about it. Have them add to their list after they have had a chance to touch and hold the object. As a class, compare the before and after observations and ask the class to classify the observations.
- Ask your students to make a list of the things they do when they are involved in an activity such as reading, writing, or problem solving. Students can share their "metacognitive" skills (learning about how one learns by self-awareness) with each other, and the class can create a list of study skills that students might want to try.
- Place ten objects on a table. Have students write as many statements as they can about how all ten are alike and how all ten are different. (Depending on the grade level of your class, you might want to use fewer objects.) Then see if students can make lists of other objects that share those similarities and differences.
- "Appearance and Reality" and "The Paradox of Changing Yet Staying the Same" make excellent focal points for philosophical discussion.

## Critical Skills Activities

- Following is a mnemonic device for a traditional, analytical, problem-solving process. The mnemonic is DALLAS.[1]

  D = Define the problem
  A = Analyze its parts
  L = List potential solutions
  L = Lop off solutions according to valid criteria, leaving two or three
  A = Analyze the remaining two or three
  S = Select a solution

  Here is a D from the story: What would be the best alternative for Light-as-a-Feather to learn how to fly? Using the story is a good introduction to the process, but the best way to involve kids in problem solving is to give them real problems, the solutions to which the students can use in their day-to-day lives.
- Divide students into teams to solve the problem discussed earlier using each step in the DALLAS process. Also evaluate the way the teams manage to cooperate and collaborate among themselves.
- Introduce criteria to evaluate the teams' organizational and leadership skills and have the teams describe the process they go through. Keep notes to compare with the next problem-solving process.
- Go through the DALLAS process a second time but shuffle the teams. Add the following: (1) Group members should ask various kinds of questions throughout the process, including content, process, and organizational questions; and (2) Individuals should gather useful information that is neatly and accurately compiled for the group to use.

## Values/Ethics Activities

### *Activity 1*

Mathew Lipman and Ann Margaret Sharp (1985) ask this question: "Can we love animals *and* eat them?" Lisa, the main character in Lipman and

1. Bloom's taxonomy is an alternative way to verify that students are using valid problem-solving processes.

Sharp's story, is confronted by a possible conflict in her own values; she is against hunting but loves to eat chicken and roast beef. Lisa's dilemma is only one of many that children face as they grow up and become aware of what produces the things, events, and habits that form their everyday lives. Following are questions you might ask students to encourage debate or as a writing assignment:

1. Can we love and hate someone at the same time? If yes, should we call our feelings love?
2. Can we love life and destroy it at the same time?
3. Since many Native Americans were slaughtered by the U.S. Cavalry, should we pay the Native Americans' descendants reparations in the form of land, housing, medical services, jobs, and democratic representation in Congress?
4. Should a mother with nine children have the right to abort a tenth pregnancy?
5. Should Union Carbide cover the complete medical costs of the Indians injured when the company released toxic poisons in India?
6. Should children have the same rights as adults?
7. Should we boycott the products of stores, companies, and corporations that pollute the environment?
8. Should we participate in government by voting?
9. Should anything be censored?
10. Should a crime involving the theft of millions of dollars by a white-collar criminal on Wall Street be considered as serious as the crimes of, say, a serial killer?

These questions may or may not be appropriate for your class, but notice that many of them begin with the word *should.* You may also choose to have groups of students brainstorm questions beginning with the word *should.* Pool the questions and have the teams discuss, share, debate, and write their opinions. You may want to conclude the activity by having each group produce a magazine with brief articles on each of the issues.

*Activity 2*

The inherent transitory quality of life prompts one to cling to it, fear its loss, and become anxious about its decay. Not only adults but teenagers and children implicitly understand life's transitory nature. There is no ethical decision that does not in some way involve the tension between holding onto and letting go of. At the heart of the struggle to create just laws is the following question: To what extent does a person's right to hold onto something infringe on someone else's right to take it away? For example, does a baker have the right to hold onto her bread if a starving person needs it to stay alive? The following activities focus on the ethical dilemma of holding onto versus letting go of.

- Read out loud the simple, moving, and wisdom-filled story *The Fall of Freddy the Leaf,* by Leo Buscaglia. While reading the story, stop four times and have your students (1) write a question and (2) comment on the story to that point. These activities will give them a reference point later as the full activity unfolds.

  When you have finished the story, gather in a circle and share the questions and the comments. After a student shares a question and a comment, have another student respond with a question, comment, or answer to the shared question.

  Next, break into three groups: the science group, the art group, and the writing group. The science group researches the organized process of the life and death of a leaf. The art group draws, paints, or sculpts renditions of a leaf. The writing group writes in various genres using the theme in the story. Put the work of the three groups together into a journal and give it a title.
- Read out loud Shel Silverstein's *The Giving Tree,* pausing as described earlier to allow children to write questions and comments. When the students break up into groups, ask each group to discuss possible answers to this question: "Should the tree have given as much as it did?" Each group should produce (1) five questions starting with "why" and an answer to the question judged most important, and (2) a letter addressed to the tree in which the students state whether or not they agree with what the tree has done.

After each group completes the tasks, have the groups share the letter. While each group is sharing their letter, members of the other groups listen and write down questions to ask after all the letters have been read. The class will hold a question-and-answer session, focusing on one group at a time. Finally, each student will write an essay or entry in a journal about what she or he has concluded in this activity.

### *A Doorway 1 Visual and Verbal Activity*

Brain processes are analogous, not digital in nature. Although Doorway 1 activities tend to be verbal and analytical, the associational or analogous nature of brain activity attracts information from the whole brain. The focus and demand of the activities behind Doorway 1 may deemphasize associated data and styles of perceiving, but such activities should never absolutely exclude data and the other styles of perceiving them. Therefore, art, music, dance, drama, movement, video, and poetry are valid pieces of the Doorway 1 puzzle as long as they serve to enhance the underlying goal of Doorway 1 processes, the establishment of cause and effect relationships between ideas and events.

### *Rube Goldberging*

Rube Goldberg was a cartoonist who satirized the encroachment of the products of technology on civilization. In creating his visual-verbal satire, he illustrated many elaborate ways to accomplish the simplest tasks. For example, if the task was to catch a fish, Goldberg might break the activity into ten or fifteen steps that would eventually result in the netting of a fish. Of course all of these steps were unnecessary elaborations intended to satirize society's increased dependence on mechanization to do even the most trivial tasks. Goldberg's satire was poignant and on target, and it gave us many humorous examples of causal relationships that are a marvelous blend of the visual and the verbal; we might call them whole-brain relationships. Figure 2.2 is a sketch similar to those of Goldberg.

For a teacher, Goldberg's work represents an idea for the teaching of the fundamental process behind Doorway 1, causal relationships. Here are the steps in an activity a teacher might assign a class:

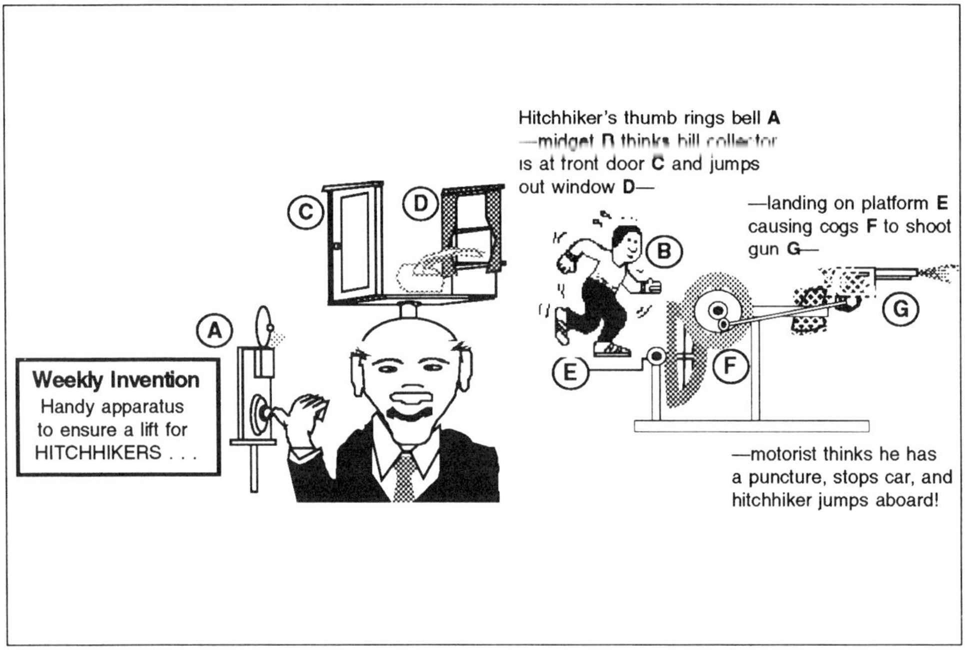

Weekly Invention
Handy apparatus to ensure a lift for HITCHHIKERS . . .
Hitchhiker's thumb rings bell **A** —midget **B** thinks bill collector is at front door **C** and jumps out window **D**—
—landing on platform **E** causing cogs **F** to shoot gun **G**—
—motorist thinks he has a puncture, stops car, and hitchhiker jumps aboard!
A
B
C
D
E
F
G


Figure 2.2. An example of a Rube Goldberg–type invention

1. Decide on a task that needs to be accomplished.
2. Think of at least ten to fifteen steps that someone could take to accomplish the task using various mechanical, electrical, chemical, and physical means. The person involved does something that represents only the first step, such as turning on a machine, after which the person is no longer involved in the process.
3. Draw the series of physical events.
4. Label the events in clearly written, sequenced, and connected steps.
5. In science class build a device that carries out the series of events and demonstrate how the device works.
6. In art class draw or paint the steps as stylishly as possible.
7. In English class, write an essay, story, or poem based on the machine.

## Atmosphere, Mood, and Brain-Wave Activity behind Doorway 1

Geoffrey and Renata Nummela Caine (1991) list two characteristics of an "optimal state of mind for meaningful learning: . . . 1. Relaxed nervous system and a sense of safety and security that operates at mental, emotional, and physical levels. 2. Student self-motivation, which is critical to the expansion of knowledge at more than surface levels" (131). To help students accomplish the work behind Doorway 1 you must become well versed in skills that enable you to create relaxed environments. If you wish to pursue analytical work with your students, you also need to develop relaxation techniques using music, color, tone of voice, body language, and guided imagery. Analytical work becomes paralyzing when divorced from the spectrum of consciousness that allows the brain to operate at slower, yet more powerful, brain-wave states that are conducive to spontaneous insights, daydreaming, and nonfocused global awareness. The rhythm between the relaxed awareness of the alpha state and the highly concentrated, externally focused beta states allows the brain to rejuvenate itself constantly.

# 3. INTUITION AND IMAGINATION

*Tests have been developed to identify creative talent. They have shown that top scorers on creativity tests averaged 23 points lower [on intelligence tests] than top scorers on [the same] intelligence tests. The most creative individuals often had trouble with problems that demanded sticking to rigid rules to find the answer.*

—Alma E. Guinness, ed.,
*Readers Digest ABC's of the Human Mind*

Doorway 2, stereotypically referred to as the "right brain," deals primarily with spatial reality, visual and auditory cues surrounding or hidden in the literate or surface dimension of objects and persons, as the objects and persons appear (such as in art) or as they participate in the process of communication (as in oral speech). Doorway 2 is the locus of dreams, inner visions, artistic insight, and what might be called the immediate apprehension of reality. These are expressed through poetry, painting, scientific breakthroughs based on hunches, and other creative endeavors.

People who use the intuition housed behind Doorway 2 develop points of view, work, writings, art, and achievements that change the world. Why? Because in spite of the enormous impact of Doorway 1 and the incredible depths to which philosophy, law, and science can reach for the good of the world, without Doorway 2 the first doorway opens to useless functional and mechanistic activity that could produce only an arid, colorless world.

In spite of the importance of intuition, however, it has been assigned a negative place in our society. Philip Goldberg (1983) states,

> The institutions that teach us how to use our minds, as well as the organizations in which we use them, are so skewed toward the rational-empirical ideal that intuition is seldom discussed, much less honored or encouraged. From grade school to graduate school, and in most of our work settings, we are taught to emulate the idealized model of scientism in our thinking, problem solving, and decision making. As a result, intuition is subject to various forms of censure and constraint. (19)

## Intuition

Peter A. Angeles (1981) defines *intuition* as follows: "Innate, instinctive knowledge or insight without the use of the sense organs, ordinary experience, or reason" (s.v. "intuition"). When we apply this definition to education, it means various things. (1) A student's exposure to curriculum can result in an understanding that initially transcends words or explanation. Teachers need to be sensitive to this phenomenon and develop ways of helping students draw out intuition in a format such as writing, art, or dialogue. (2) Curricula need not always be organized in logical, sequential terms since understanding is not necessarily dependent on logical, sequential arrangements. (3) Intuition does not bypass the senses, but it bypasses those parts of the senses that serve merely as receptors of external data. Teachers can tap the intuitive senses by helping students focus inward—on feelings, images, visions, and sensations—and helping students to bring forth such inner workings.

Goldberg (1983) describes the importance of the relationship between rational inquiry and intuition:

> Only when abstract concepts are truly *known,* apprehended with direct intuitive intimacy, can they take on the kind of experiential quality that can transform behavior. We protect and nurture that

> which we perceive as part of ourselves, but the sense of connection with people and nature has to be deeply felt, not just thought about. Furthermore, while certain beliefs can foster a willingness to act responsibly, they don't tell us how to do it or what the consequences of specific actions will be. For this we need intuition. (215)

Goldberg's observation raises the following practical questions for teachers: (1) Do we see teaching as merely the transmission of information and data? Or is teaching the act of helping students understand, so that in some way their lives are changed by the information they take in? (2) Can we create activities that allow the intuitive selves of students to rise to the surface, grab data, and bring that data back into the students' depths, thereby making the knowledge real? (3) Because knowledge is about the self, others, and the world and how all of them are interrelated, is the primary role of the teacher *to help children imagine, feel, and sense what they know?*

Frances E. Vaughan (1979) characterizes intuition partly as a kind of inner teacher that gives us all kinds of information that is true. She states, "The willingness to follow the guidance of this inner teacher is trusting intuition. Behind fear, anger, depression, and anxiety is hidden the capacity for love, joy, serenity, and compassion. Behind all emotions is the wisdom of intuition that can lead one to the full experience of the central core of being. The more you are willing to open yourself to the full awareness that is potentially yours, the more authentically you can live your life" (176).

What are the implications of this statement for teachers? First, learning involves taking risks, a willingness to trust. Too much emphasis on Doorway 1 erodes risk taking because the very nature of logic is to exhaust all terms and all sequences. When we are operating from Doorway 1, we never jump from A to Z; we travel the safe, linear path through all the letters in between. Intuitive learning involves a leap of faith into the inner self, where one finds quite clearly what one knows and senses about what is happening "out there." Second, intuition personalizes learning by appealing to an inner, cogitating self that understands more than the externally oriented cogitating self of Doorway 1. Finally, the role of the teacher is to help students feel comfortable opening up to their inner lives and to the idea that their inner selves have a right to understand and mold whatever the students come across in their own wonderful ways. To do so, teachers must first value their own inner lives.

Vaughan also states, "If you are serious about wanting to fully experience the potential of both the right and left hemispheres of the brain and find a lifestyle that is truly satisfying to you, then you must give yourself the time and space necessary for allowing your intuition to come into conscious awareness. Remember, there is nothing you can do to make intuition happen, but there is much you can do to allow it to happen" (176–77). Again, what practical consequences does Vaughan's observation have for teachers? (1) Students need a truly whole-brain approach that taps the intuitive domain. (2) Students need intuition to appreciate causation fully. (3) To help students live in a self-fulfilling manner, teachers must help students trust the students' intuitions and hunches. (4) Teachers cannot teach intuition, but they can provide specific activities that will allow intuition to surface.

## Allowing Intuition to Surface

### *Activity 1*

Make sure students have paper and pens on their desks. While playing Pachelbel's Canon in D in the background, ask your students to sit facing a window that is open to the outdoors and, preferably, to the sky. Explain to your students that you would like them to let the music and the scene from the window carry them away into a daydream. Every so often you will interrupt this dreaminess with questions you would like them to respond to in writing. Allow two to three minutes to pass before having them respond to one of the following:

- Explain how you feel.
- Imagine you are an eagle flying across the sky. Describe what you see.
- What colors do you feel like right now?
- Write a statement about the universe that you don't think you've made before.
- Write about who you are in a way you may not have written at any other time.

You will need to adapt these directions to the grade level of your students. For example, the last two directions may be too abstract for early elementary grades. The following may be adequate substitutes:

- Can you write something or draw something that shows how you feel about our home, the Earth?
- Can you write something that the music and your daydream make you feel about someone you love?

*Activity 2*

While playing *At the Edge* by Mickey Hart ask your students to doodle and write on a large piece of paper whatever thoughts come to their minds, as if they were creating graffiti on a building. Continue the activity for 5 to 10 minutes. Then ask students to redraw the graffiti or draw the thought they are most interested in. Lastly, have them make posters of their drawings and write essays explaining the thoughts. Play music that produces a reverie. Display all the works around the room. Have students roam the room as if it were a museum, taking notes on each combination of the visual and verbal.

When you have completed activities 1 and 2, have a "debriefing" session in which the students make observations, ask questions, and answer your questions. If the activities were successful, you will notice the fruits of intuitive and imaginative release for a long time, especially if you make such a focus part of the pattern of your class.

John Curtis Gowan (1974) suggests that intuition is that part of the preconscious life that is available to the conscious mind. He states that our "species wide intelligence is embedded in the preconscious of each of us" (7). Gowan goes on to list the characteristics of this preconsciousness:

1. It is a unity, a plenum.
2. It exists in a state of complete suggestibility.
3. It has complete memory of all matters, past, present, and future.
4. It is able to control, maintain, and safeguard the body and its health.
5. It produces phantasms of the living or dead or the content of dreams.
6. It influences conditions and events.

Gowan also discusses the conditions under which the preconscious and conscious minds merge. Among these conditions Gowan lists "trance states and in certain conditions spontaneous disassociated states" (8). Teachers can use these trance states in the classroom to help students learn. A trance state results when an experience holds all attention, forcing a person to put critical faculties of judgment on hold. Following is a list of situations where people, young or old, enter normal trance states:

1. While listening to speeches, sermons, and advertising pitches
2. While looking at art in museums
3. While walking on the beach or strolling anywhere that the natural environment produces a sense of peace, wonder, and awe
4. Just before going to sleep and just after awakening
5. While daydreaming
6. While listening to music
7. While shopping
8. While doing repetitive or ritualized work, such as cooking a meal or driving a car to and from work
9. During all peak experiences
10. During learning experiences that engage the learner totally

Many experts believe that children up to about seven years of age are enveloped in trances that make fairy tales, goblins, and elves seem real to them. While in these trance states, the children externalize many of their story experiences, so their universe is not as rationally compartmentalized and composed of spatially separated entities as adults' universe. If you have ever watched children who are listening to stories, you have seen them in these trance states. In fact, stories, myths, and fairy tales help children begin to come to terms with their preconscious minds, a process that should flower into a lifetime of conscious creative living. For teachers, knowledge of this trance state leads to one question: *What can I do to tap this inner awareness without the energy, power, and knowingness of this region getting out of hand because I either release too much of it too soon or don't help release enough of it at the right time?* You can tap this awareness by exposing your students to stories across the curriculum, beginning in kindergarten and continuing through high school. Fairy tales work especially well for young students.

Bruno Bettelheim (1977) discusses the role fairy tales play in the lives of children:

> Some unconscious pressures in children can be worked out through play. But many do not lend themselves to it because they are too complex and contradictory or too dangerous and socially disapproved. Here, knowing fairy tales is a great help to the child, as illustrated by the fact that many fairy stories are acted out by children, but only after the children have become familiar with the story which they could never have invented on their own. (55)

We might say that the storage house of a child's experiences, and of all people's experiences, really, is so vast that it requires a filter that opens more and more, depending on the individual's needs and capacity to deal with this vastness. For children the symbolic filter of the fairy tale is perfect. It is one of the earliest forms of literature that teachers need to master if they are to commit themselves to allowing the intuitive, preconscious process in children to grow and develop as it must for mental, physical, and intellectual development.

## A Fairy Tale Activity in the Intuitive Domain

Bettelheim notes further that the more familiar students become with a story, the easier each child can externalize the meaning of the story, implicitly externalizing their own preconscious awareness and intuitive powers of analysis. Bettelheim warns against rushing too quickly from one fairy tale to another. He suggests instead you gently engage children in responding to and searching thoroughly through one tale.

### *Materials*

- Copy of Grimm's "Hansel and Gretel"
- Copy of Bruno Bettelheim's commentary on "Hansel and Gretel" from *The Uses of Enchantment* (159–66)
- Art supplies: crayons and art paper, possibly paints, scissors, and glue
- Relaxing music
- Camcorder, VCR, and TV

*Doing the Activity*

1. Set up the camcorder and arrange to have someone videotape the activity from start to finish, including all the preparations students make.
2. While you are setting up and organizing, play soft music in the background. *Shoreline* by David Blonski with Synchestra would work well (Elfin Music Co., Box 915, Camden, Mass. 04843).
3. Depending on the size of your classroom, divide the class into small groups and give them paper, pens, crayons, paints, and scissors.
4. If you are working with younger students, review the plot of "Hansel and Gretel": ask for details of the plot and for the reasons the children think the tale was written.
5. If the children have not heard the tale, introduce it by asking, "What would you say, think, feel, or imagine if someone told you a story about . . . ?" Draw the children out as much as you can.
6. Read halfway through the story.
7. Ask the children to repeat what has happened so far.
8. Take a short break and interview a few children; ask them how they feel about the story.
9. Read the rest of the story.
10. Ask the children to do any of the following:

    Draw a character or scene from the story and explain why they chose that character or scene.

    Take paints and fill a canvas with colors that represent how the story makes them feel.

    Write a letter to a character in the story being sure to express how they feel about that character.

    Create masks of the characters, cut the masks out, tape or glue them to a stick, and, with others, reenact parts of the story.

In teams of at least three, create questions about the story, being sure to have many of them start with "why" and "should." Use the questions as the basis for a large group discussion.

Joseph Chilton Pearce can deepen our understanding of intuition. Pearce (1985) refers to the development of the mid-brain's (limbic system's) role in mediating between the lower brain (reticular system) and the higher brain (neocortical system). He writes of the aborigine's idea of Dream Time to develop his point:

> The aborigine believe[s] that every man, woman, animal, blade of grass, water hole, or tree ha[s] a counterpart, a subtle or dream image. The plan of the world is laid out in this dream form and enacted now, in the physical world. A perfect coordination and cooperation with Dream Time assures [humans] a perfect relation with the form which shapes our world, with creation itself. Dream time refers to the general blueprint out of which life springs. *Intuition is our innate capacity for becoming aware of this subtle energy as needed for our biological well being.* (70; emphasis added)

Pearce tells us that this subtle energy blossoms between the ages of four and seven and that, if the powers of intuition do not develop at this time "through proper modeling and guidance, the possibility for such action generally atrophies, as the weight of attention shifts to the new blueprint" (68).

Although the ages for developing intuition may be more flexible than Pearce's theory suggests, one thing is certain: Intuition is a real, fundamental power of the mind by which human beings, even at very early ages, make contact with something enormously powerful at the heart of the universe and gradually bring it into being. The first manifestation of this power is through some form of imagery.

## Imagination

Although we may have a stereotypical view of scientists as hyperlogical, Einstein emphasized the importance of imagination as a premium source of scientific discovery. Many educators are not familiar with Einstein's perspective, nor with Edgar Allen Poe's view of the importance of imagination in our thought processes.

In Poe's piece titled, "Eureka: An Essay on the Material and Spiritual Universe," he comments on the role intuition and imagination play in scientific exploration. Through the guise of a fictional character in the year 2848, Poe (1904) writes the following:

> You can easily understand how restrictions so absurd on their very face must have operated, in those days, to retard the progress of true Science, which makes its most important advances—as all History will show—by seemingly intuitive leaps. These ancient ideas confined investigating to crawling; and I need not suggest to you that crawling, among varieties of locomotion, is a very capital thing of its kind; but because the tortoise is sure of foot, for this reason must we clip the wings of eagles? (11)

Continuing to speak through this fictional character, Poe pokes fun at the narrow scientific reasoning of many by pointing out that Newton deduced the law of gravity based on work done by Kepler, who *guessed* at the laws he proclaimed:

> Yes, these vital laws Kepler guessed—that is to say he imagined them. Had he been asked to point out either the deductive or inductive route by which he attained them, his reply might have been—"I know nothing about routes—but I do know the machinery of the universe. Here it is. I grasped it with my soul—I reached it through mere hint of intuiting." (11)

In another essay, "Colloquy of Monos and Una," Poe (1904) describes the connection between music and imagination. He contended that the qualities of music (poetic diction, sentiment, and creation) are those that speak directly to the soul, to the intuitive imagination.

## An Activity that Speaks to the Imagination

### *Materials*

Any of the following:

Any Windham Hill album
Dvorak Symphony No. 9 from *The New World*
*Passages* by Ravi Shankar and Philip Glass
*Watermark* by Enya
*Meditations* by Yusef Lateef
*Brahm's Violin Concerto* with Nigel Kennedy
*You Think You Know Me* by Ezra Ngcukana

Drawing and composition paper, pencils, pens, crayons, paints
Handouts listing the music selections

A handout with the sets of eyes as described below:

*The Activity*

1. Cut out pictures of ten to twelve well-known people from magazines, newspapers, or other sources. List the people whose pictures you have cut out and assign them each a letter, *a* through *j* or *l*. Then cut out their eyes in sets, being sure to cut any other features away from the eyes. You can keep the eyes separate or paste them onto one sheet of paper and copy them, depending on how you choose to do the next step. Be sure to identify the eyes in some way so that you know whom they belong to. You may want to keep the pictures so you can piece them back together at the end of the activity.
2. Hand out pictures of the eyes or place them on a table where all students can see them. Do not tell students whom the eyes belong to. While you play music in the background, students will study the sets of eyes quietly. After a few minutes, each student will select four sets of eyes that he or she feels something for.
3. Give students writing and art supplies. Students will write about what kind of people they think their four sets of eyes belong to. Emphasize that students should develop their sense of the person and express that sense in as elaborate a way as possible.
4. Have each student select two sets of eyes from those he or she has not already used. The first set should be one that the student feels belongs to someone who may be capable of criminal activity. The second set should be of the person that the student senses is compassionate and considerate of others. From among the six selections (four that said something to her or him and the two that she or he has characterized), each student will pick one set and draw or paint what he or she thinks the rest of the person looks like. Be sure that students can tell what in the eyes made them draw or paint their pictures as they did.

5. Turn off the music and ask students to share comments about each set of eyes. When students have finished, reveal the identity of the person behind each set of eyes. Discuss the surprises, accurate readings, and descriptions of the people behind the eyes.

The combination of the music, the mystery of the eyes, and the hidden identity forces a certain degree of nonlinear thought that hooks associations, hunches, feelings, sensations, and intuitions about the eyes. This kind of activity can build intuition and imaginative thought, especially when you play the music to stir the imaginative soul into another realm of thinking.

Hannah Arendt (1978), a philosopher, writer, and educator, reminds us that "the [verb] 'to know' is a derivative of the [verb] 'to see.' To see is *idein* (in the Greek), to know is *eidenai,* that is, to have seen. First you see, then you know" (87). All knowing, according to Arendt, is bound up with both outer vision, sight, and inner vision, imagination. She states, "By repeating in imagination, we *de-sense* whatever had been given to our senses. And only in this immaterial form can our thinking faculty now begin to concern itself with these data" (87). In other words, the operations of thought behind Doorway 1 are utterly dependent on the sensation and imagination behind Doorway 2.

Arendt (1978) reminds us that in China, thought is expressed in images, not words. Chinese script embodies the visual symbols of what it is stating so that "Poetry even to read aloud, will affect the hearer[s] optically; [they] will not stick to the word [they] hear but to the sign [they] remember and with it to the sights to which the sign clearly points" (101). In the West we abstract from experience to produce words that are, theoretically, not monograms or pictographs of the original experience, yet they stimulate a representation of the object in the imagination. Arendt concludes that East and West do share the "unique/toned priority of vision for mental activities" (101). Her definition of imagination follows: "Re-presentation, making present what is actually absent, is the mind's unique gift, and drawn from vision's experience, this gift is called imagination" (76).

Maxine Greene (1988) states quite clearly that "For Dewey, experience becomes fully conscious only when meanings derived from earlier experience enter in through the exercise of the imaginative capacity" (125). The importance of imagination lies in its uncertainty and in its very nature, unfixed and untamed by specific ideologies, codes, and goals. In the framework of teaching it is what makes learning free, exciting, and self-discovering. It is self-discovery not in the sense of a narcissistic pandering to the self, but rather self-discovery based on the freedom to think, discover, express, and form one's own thoughts.

Greene (1978) also speaks of the centrality of the arts in evoking imagination: "To engage authentically with a painting, a ballet, a musical work, we must—by dint of imaginative activity—be released into our own streams of consciousness, our own inner time" (199). Remember the aborigine's Dream Time? Is this not the same as "our own inner time"? Is not Doorway 2 the doorway into Dream Time, inner time, imagination, intuition, and the stream of all streams of consciousness? Is this not also why we can say that Doorway 2 is the portal into the outer space and art that one first experiences with the five senses and into the inner space or the locus of art that one experiences with corresponding inner senses?

## The Art of Inner Space

Inner space is a location *within* the boundaries of our skin. It is unimportant to define the location of inner space as the repository of the soul or as the house of the spirit. All the experiences of inner space as I refer to them here are as physical in nature as those experiences that involve interactions with people, places, and things external to the skin.

The art of inner space is primarily the uncontrolled contact we have with sensory images, be they visual, auditory, gustatory, tactile, olfactory, kinesthetic, or synesthetic, without reference to the outside world. Art at this level is created in the dream first and foremost. At this primary level one can self-induce all of the above types of images while dreaming or while awake. Self-induced manipulation of the primary art of inner space, dream imagery, involves lucid dreaming, awareness that one is dreaming, and the ability to enter one's own dream to rearrange things.

Technology has externalized inner space into a cybernetic illusion called "virtual reality." Virtual reality is, in essence, inner space mimed by technology. Because virtual reality will become an enormous force in society, it is vital to distinguish it from true inner space so that children can still tap into their own inner space without depending too much on the technological representation of it.

The secondary level of the art of inner space involves some contact with an external stimulus such as a story, music, or another sensation. The outer reality serves the art of inner space. One might describe the outer reality as the original fuel that launches a rocket that will eventually orbit the Earth and, to a great extent, leave behind what it was that got it there. Some refer to this as guided imagery or visualization. As Maureen Murdock (1987) says,

> Guided imagery is a process of going within, focusing attention on breath and bodily relaxation and moving to deeper levels of consciousness where more images are accessible to the conscious mind. This may take the form of a pleasant journey to the beach or mountains, a meeting with an inner figure of wisdom, or visualizing yourself in whatever field of endeavor is your focus. Each time I lead an imagery exercise I learn something new about the infinite possibilities for learning, healing and creativity with this technique. (2–3)

Beverly-Colleene Galyean introduced me to visualization in 1981 using a visualization called "The Rose." It was so moving that I have used it in all grade levels, from early elementary through adult education. I must state emphatically that visualization will become one of the most powerful, effective, and necessary tools for teachers in the years to come. Harnessing inner space will revolutionize teaching and learning. Although most teachers have heard of the technique, the majority of them don't use it. But we must use it as an essential and basic teaching skill.

## The Visualization Process

Visualization technique is connected to relaxation and slows brain-wave processes to the speed of stronger, higher-amplitude alpha waves. What follows are the steps in the process, including the actual guided-imagery journey and post-visualization activities for all levels.

### *Step 1: The Explanation*

Explain to the students that they are going on an inner journey involving their ability to imagine. Inform them that with their eyes closed they will listen to you describe a journey, a scene, or a situation, and they can write about, create art about, and share the experience with others. Ask them to relax, follow your directions, listen carefully, and follow the inner experience as it unfolds.

*Step 2: The Relaxation*

Students should be sitting or lying down in a comfortable position with their eyes closed. Draw their attention to their breathing, especially the change in temperature from cool inhale to warmer exhale. Spend some time concentrating on this rhythm. Next focus on the heartbeat and the rhythm or pulse that it produces through the body. Ask students to scan their bodies to sense this rippling pulse. Spend some time helping them focus on this pulse, then announce the guided journey is about to begin.

*Step 3: The Rose*

Read the following, which is an adaptation of Galyean's visualization, to your students.

*Imagine yourself at the opening to a forest on a sunny, mildly breezy day in summer. The sky is blue. You begin to walk the path through the forest trying to notice everything around you: the trees, the birds, the sound of your feet, the smell of the pine-scented fresh air, and the taste of a piece of mint leaf you've picked and placed in your mouth.*

*As you continue along the path, you notice how the sunlight is sliced into many long, narrow sheets of transparent and luminescent air. You hear the sound of rabbits and other small creatures scurrying through the fallen twigs and brush that accumulate in a forest. The path rises a bit and to the right you see a large rock and behind it a cave, but you don't stop until the path comes to a small footbridge that crosses a stream. Before crossing, you carefully work your way down to the stream, listen attentively to its flow, catch your reflection in its crystal clear waters, and dip your hands into its coolness, bringing up to your face a splash of refreshment that causes your mouth to smile and your heart to pick up the beat. You leave the stream, cross the old wooden bridge and continue along the path until it ends at an opening to a large field of tall meadow grass of green and yellow.*

*You are awash with sunlight, unprotected by the long shadows of tall trees, and you walk through the tall weedy grass, feeling it tickle your hands and wrists, until you notice ahead of you a small hill that is flat at the top and that, from a distance, seems to be a garden of some sort. You make your way to the hill, feeling the gentle breeze cool you and bend the tall grass. At the bottom of the hill you pause for breath and begin to climb.*

*When you arrive at the top of the hill you see before you one of the most beautiful flower gardens you have ever seen. The flowers explode with color and fill the air with the sweetest perfume. All the multicolored flowers are arranged in a circle, and in the middle a single, vibrant, red rose stands tall above all the others as if it were the king or queen of the garden. You watch the red rose and sense that it is calling to you; you slowly walk toward it, careful not to step on any of the flowers. When you reach the rose, you kneel down next to it. It whispers to you that if you like, you too may become a red rose in this magic garden. It assures you that you will be a rose for only a few seconds and that, when the time is up, you will return to your human form. You agree to take the opportunity.*

*As you become a rose, the first thing you feel is how deep your roots go into the ground, as if the Earth were hugging you to make you feel safe and secure. When the breeze blows, you have no fear of breaking because you have the power to bend in the wind, and the wind tickles your petals and whispers love songs to you. The sun feels warm and the energy it fills you with makes you happy and strong. A bee comes to land within you and you hear the hum of its wings echo between your petals; you see the bee smile and say thank you. A rain cloud forms in the sky, and rain falls upon you and the ground you are rooted in. It is refreshingly cool and playful. You are content just being there, for as a rose in the garden you are at peace and in harmony with the rest of nature.*

*It dawns on you that your time as a rose is nearly up and you spend some time appreciating this momentary gift. You feel yourself return to your human shape, kneeling before the single rose in the garden, now understanding firsthand what it is like to be a flower. You rise to your feet, walk to the edge of the garden, and say goodbye to all the flowers, especially to the single red rose in the middle. Just as you turn to retrace your steps to where your journey began, you hear all the flowers chant softly to you: "You have the power, you have the power!"*

*Walking down the hill through the field of tall grass to the opening into the forest, you ponder the message of the flowers. You walk into the forest, over the footbridge, past the gurgling stream, noticing the large rock and cave to your left and promising yourself that you will return to the cave some day. As your path leads you back to where your journey began, you begin to smile, for you think you understand what the flowers meant. The path ends and you step out from it into your regular life; maybe you are at school, maybe you are at home, maybe you are where you play, maybe you are at a relative's house, or maybe you are back a long time ago when magic and wonder filled the Earth and the lion and the lamb sat down with each other to share their stories and to give each other flowers.*

*Step 4: The Return*

When the journey is over, tell the children that they may open their eyes slowly and that they might like to do so while you count backward from 10 to 1. Many find it comforting to listen to appropriately dreamy music.

*Step 5: The Immediate Writing Exercise*

Regardless what age group or what discipline you use the visualization for, it is important that the students free write about the event. They should write for as long as it takes them to empty onto paper what the journey was and what the journey meant to them. Remind them that each student's journey was different because each person's mind and imagination added things that made the journey unique. Ask them to reflect on what they saw, felt, heard, tasted, and smelled on their journey. Last, ask them to reflect on the chanted message of the flowers as well as the curious cave. Focusing on the cave will prepare them for a visualization in which they return to the cave and explore it. Such a focus allows one visualization to link with others that follow.

*Step 6. Drawing or Painting*

When students have explored their ideas as fully as possible through writing, it is time for art. Ask the students to pick a medium (pencil, crayon, paint, and so on) and draw the rose, taking into account the roses they had become. You might ask them to draw two roses, one with each hand, then ask them to compare the pictures. Did one rose feel better as they drew it or did one rose have a quality the other did not? You might see some qualitative differences that reflect lateralization of the brain.

*Step 7: A Second Writing Exercise*

Beneath the drawn or painted rose, ask children to write some text on "What It Means to Be a Rose." You can display the artwork and written responses.

*Step 8: Rewrite of the "Immediate Write"*

Ask students to rewrite and edit their original responses, making the pieces as perfect as they can in terms of spelling, grammar, sentence structure, vocabulary, and so on.

*Step 9: Reading*

As part of a whole-language approach at the early elementary level, you may choose to make booklets of the writings and pass the booklets out as reading material for the class. Use the booklets to explore the specific phonic or vocabulary skills you think important. In higher grades, you may have students compile booklets and share them, read them aloud, and discuss them or simply read them in a peer editing process.

*Step 10: Discussion*

Have students write questions about the journey and let these questions be the basis for a discussion.

## Using Guided Imagery across the Curriculum

Beverly-Colleene Galyean (1983) takes us through spelling, language arts, social studies, mathematics, and science to prove the usefulness of what she terms "guided cognitive imageries." We know that firsthand experience forms the best basis for all learning. Because visualization produces real experience, a student may use visualization to enrich a journey through any of the disciplines. We must count the experience of inner space among the most primary, basic, and effective experiential starting places for all learning. Following are some quick suggestions for using guided imagery across the curriculum:

*Science*

- Take your students on a swim with the fish and undersea life around the world.
- Take the children through the growth cycle of a leaf.
- Take the children through the Amazon rain forest by having them become animals or insects indigenous to the area.

*Mathematics*

- Have students imagine geometrical shapes and visualize building structures with them.
- Imagine numbers and the process of addition and subtraction.
- Read word problems slowly while students have their eyes open and while students have their eyes shut.

*Spelling*

- While playing baroque music that has sixty beats per minute, read through a list of words.
- Go through the list of words again and ask children to draw the letters simultaneously in the air.
- Ask each child to recite each of the words and spell it aloud.

*Language Arts*

- Have students write an "I Am" poem from a visualization experience, suggesting that they use the stream of internal images to produce the "I Am" identifications. Be sure the descriptions go beyond the simple identification with the inner image.
- Develop a mnemonic that requires students to visualize a clue as the bridge between a word and its meaning, for example, "alacrity" means "speed" and a student could visualize "alac the turtle" who possessed "a lac(k)" of speed.
- In a guided imagery, take the kids to a campfire in a cave where they meet a wise person who gives them a gift.

Language arts teachers talk about the "authentic voice" that people use to write from themselves and that results in a unique "voice print." Guided imagery journeys and subsequent free-writing periods produce this authentic voice.

## The Art of Outer Space

Although there exists no territorial boundary between inner space and outer space, we can use the term *outer space* to mean the open-eyed creation or use of an external form that our senses appreciate. The following activities require students to produce or use external images in order to write and read with greater interest, skill, and comprehension.

## The Mandala Experience

The word *mandala* means "circle." It has come to represent any circular expression of the self either drawn, painted, sculpted, or danced. The use of the mandala comes from Tibetan culture and found its way to the West through the work of Carl Jung. Jung used the mandala to develop his self-understanding and the healing process of his patients and noted that the mandala occurs in various cultures, such as the Native American "medicine wheel," and even in our fascination with what he called the "rotundum" or circular shape of the UFO.

In psychological terms, the mandala expresses either a sense of wholeness or those things or events that prevent wholeness, that is, those things that have fractured the wholeness and that we seek to express and understand as the path toward the reunification of the self. We know that the word *education* comes from the Latin *educare,* "to lead out from within." Education is thus an activity in which the self creates an expression of itself and simultaneously takes in information to nourish this eventual cyclic return to expression of the self. The mandala fits perfectly into this cyclic activity that is at the heart of education. If you use the mandala well in your school activities, you will influence your students' reading, writing, and thinking enormously.

### *A Possible Way to Start*

Judith Cornell (1990) has developed an activity called "Creating a Simple Color Wheel" (55–60). In this activity, a person draws a circle and divides it into twelve equal pieces. In each piece the person fills in a color, tone, or hue to create a feeling and an appreciation of color. This activity is a good way to introduce children to making mandalas. You can follow the activity with a discussion of how the color wheel makes your students feel.

Maureen Murdock (1987) does a visualization exercise in which students visualize a circle that eventually encompasses the whole universe. When she has finished the visualization, she has students cut out a cardboard wheel and begin making mandalas (95). This activity is another excellent way to glide into the mandala experience.

Beverly-Colleene Galyean (1983) uses the same approach as Maureen Murdock except Galyean asks the child to pay attention to the "colors, textures, images, symbols, lines, various shapes going from us at the center to all areas of the mind" (174). She follows the visualization with a mandala-making exercise.

*A Step-by-Step Approach*

Following is a sequential activity that leads to the creation of a mandala that is at once harmonious, geometrically balanced, and filled with imagination and intuitive expression:

1. Explain the word *mandala*.
2. Have students draw a circle and divide it into quarters, as in the following picture.

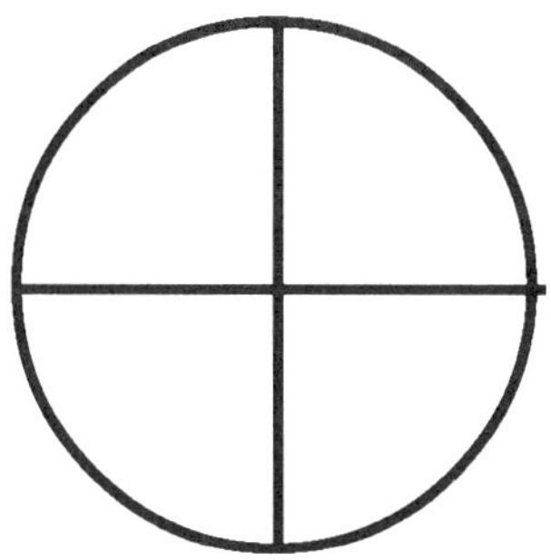

3. Have students draw concentric circles in the larger circle.

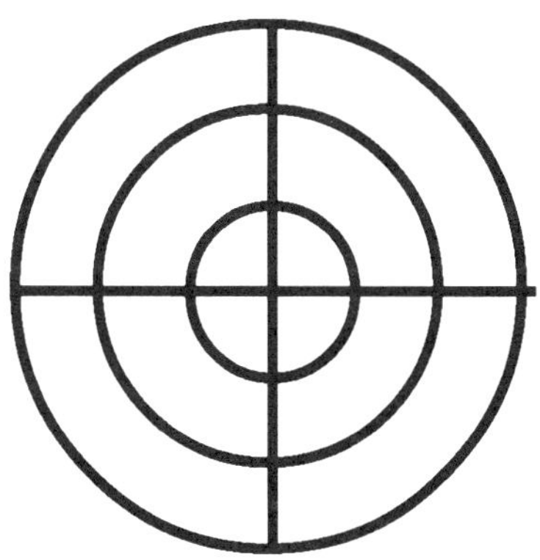

4. Tell students the rule of balance, which is creating mirror images of the top and bottom halves or the left and right halves. Students can also mirror diagonally; for example, if the student mirrors the top and bottom halves and the top left corner differs from the top right corner, the top left quarter may be mirrored by the right bottom quarter, as in the following picture:

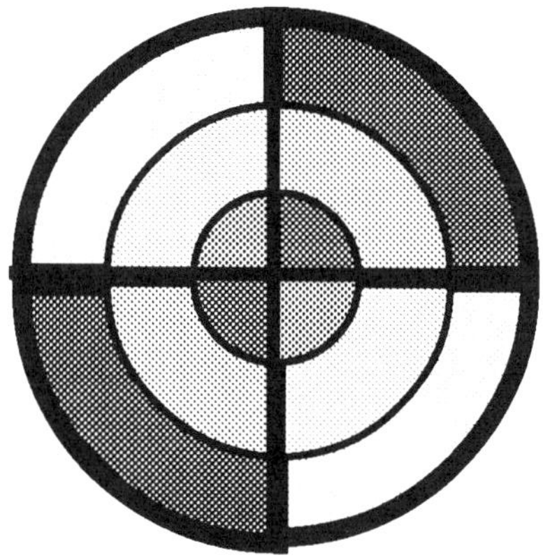

5. Explain to students that making mandalas takes time and that the children should create the designs slowly, peacefully, and very carefully.
6. Have students name their mandalas, for example, "The Mandala of Future Vision" or "The Mandala of Love."
7. You may follow the activity with poetry, essays, stories, or dialogues that each student finds or writes that inspire and reflect his or her mandala.

*The Mandala as a Study Guide*

You can use mandalas across the curriculum as a way to help students remember the material they have read. Each student fills each concentric circle in the four quadrants with information from any reading assignment in science, social studies, or language arts books. The mandala becomes a visual cue that triggers associations between what students have read and their values.

Following are examples of high school ESL students' mandalas. The teacher took one of my mandala-making workshops. You will notice the harmony and balance in each mandala and that the activity evoked not only the students' feelings but also a sense of caring for what they did.

*Mandala of Life*

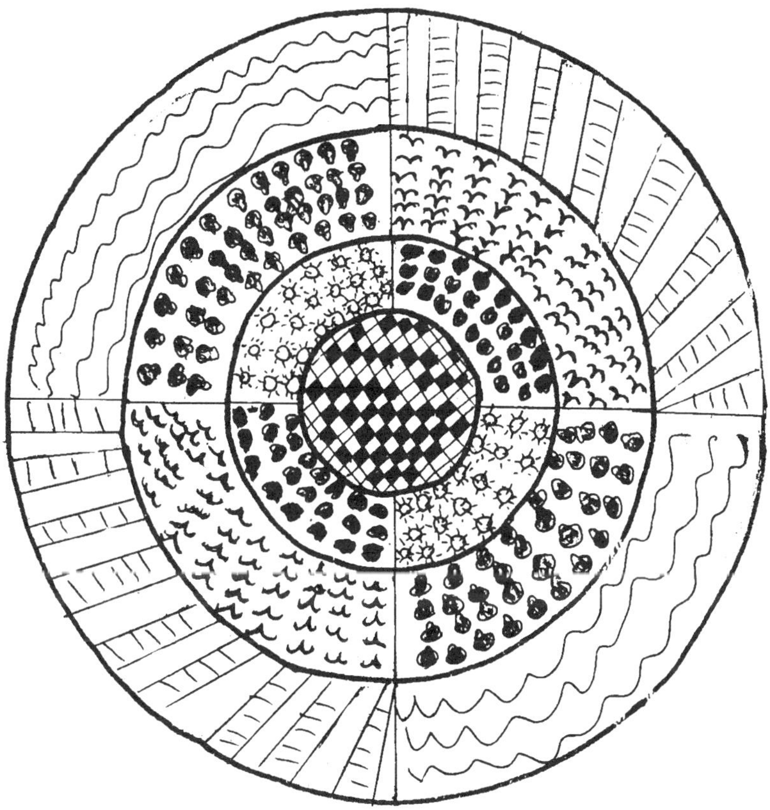

In my Mandala the hearts represent love because love is full of the world. The sun represents that we live because of the sun. In the world parts I have birds that represent peace and skeleton bones that represent war. Finally in the dreams part the waves represent dreams because they are easy to forget.

*The Mandala of Dreams*

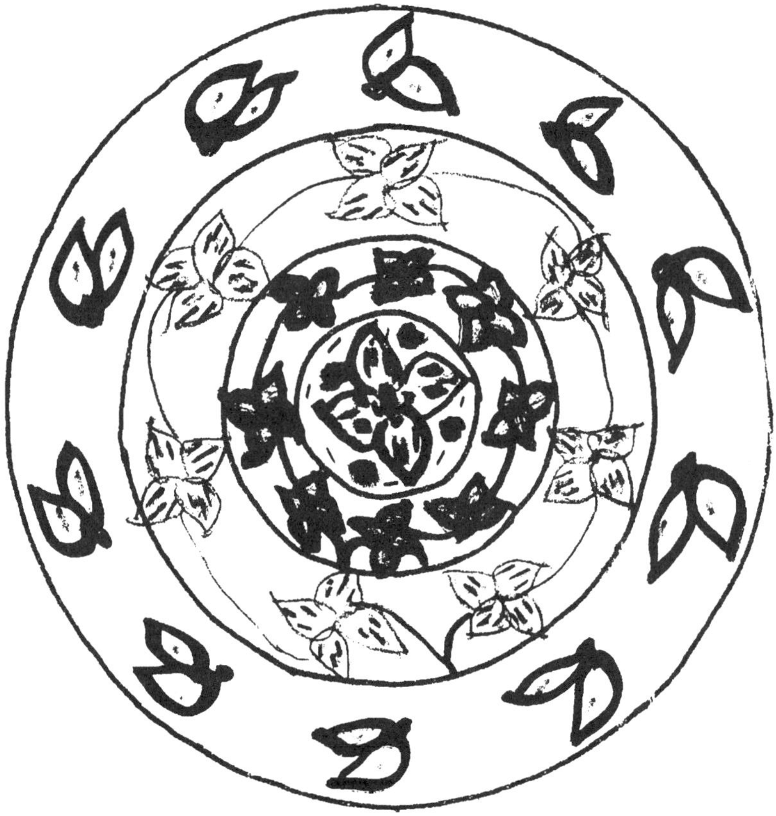

I think my Mandala is a world of dreams. The flowers on the Mandala are like my dreams. I hope my dreams come true. Everywhere there are flowers. No one is sad. Everybody is happy in all the world. Beautiful birds and bees fly and play with the flowers.

*The Mandala of Love, Hope, and Honesty*

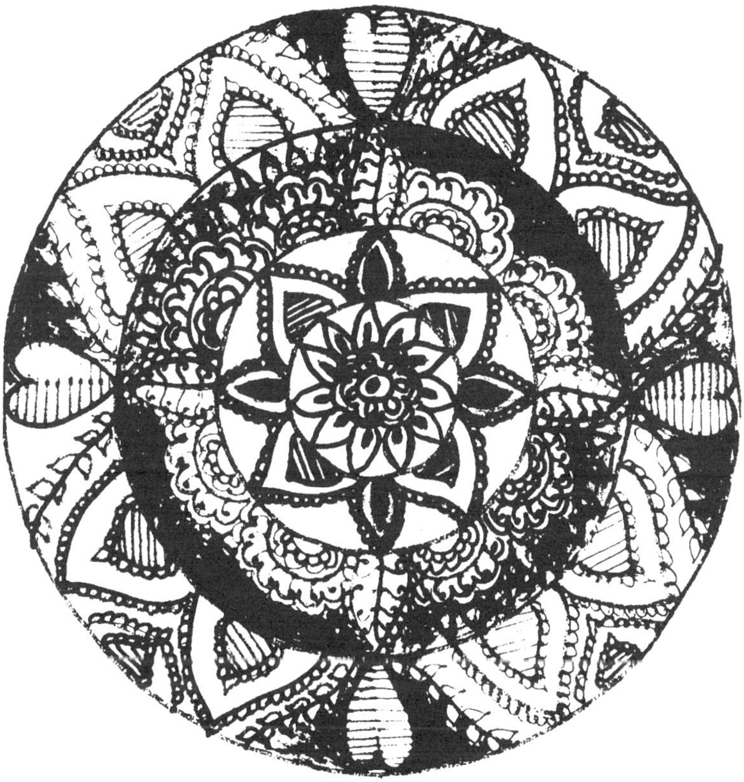

In my world I drew leaves because leaves are green and the color of green is cold. This means my world's people are nice. I drew a design of tiny circles because I have so many dreams that they don't fit into my circles. I tried to fill them. In every tiny design are my hopes. . . . I drew a heart in my love circles because my heart is very big. In my heart everybody can live. My heart is for those people who have love, hope and honesty. "Honesty is the best policy."

## Abstract Designs, Viewing, Reading, and Writing

Abstract design is another art form that reflects outer space. By abstract design I mean any visual form drawn for or used to express or comprehend some meaning.

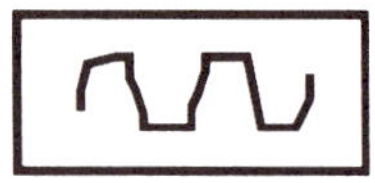

This simple design could mean many things, such as the rhythm of life, the notion of slow but sure, beginnings and endings, and many other things. One might draw such a design to express a feeling, an idea, or as a symbol for something one viewed on TV or read in a book. As you study the abstract design activities, you will realize what the designs are and that they are powerful tools of expression and comprehension across the curriculum.

### *Abstract Designs and Cartoons*

For this activity you might watch a series of cartoons having some theme in mind, such as relationships. Your students would watch one cartoon, complete the response outlined below, and move on through any number of cartoons appropriate for the age of your students and the amount of time you want to spend on the activity. The object of the activity is for students to use cartoons to advance thinking skills behind Doorway 1 by using the intuitive skills housed behind Doorway 2.

Give each student a copy of the following chart of abstract designs:

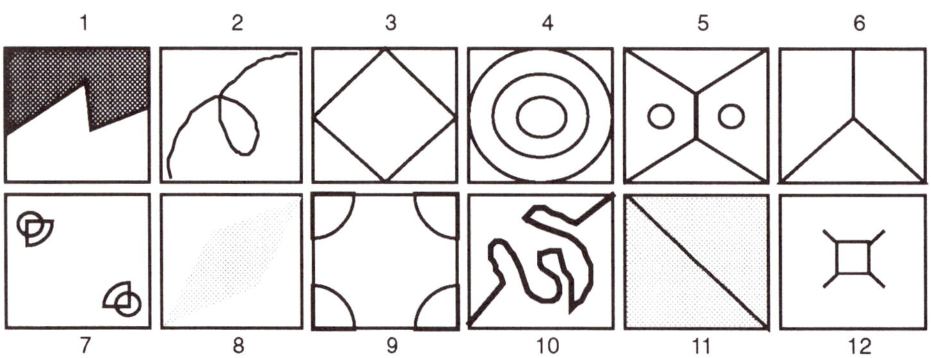

After watching cartoon 1, each student selects the design that best represents what relationships were like in the cartoon. Then the student writes a brief explanation of why she or he selected the design.

Repeat this process for all the cartoons you have selected, then have students share their selections and explanations. You can develop a larger assignment from this activity, such as "How Cartoons Depict Relationships."

### *Abstract Designs and Reading*

You can use abstract designs to enhance reading comprehension. After your students have read a poem, short story, novel, or textbook selection, they select an abstract design to represent what they read and they explain the selection. Gradually, the students create their own designs and explain the link.

### *Abstract Designs and Writing*

Select a design based on its thematic or aesthetic value or have your students select the design and have them write about it.

### *Abstract Designs and Theme Making*

Collect twenty to thirty designs and put them on a large piece of paper. With your students, list the themes expressed in the designs (love, greed, joy, beauty, and so on) and match the designs with the themes they express. Create groups, placing students who make the same matches in one group. The students discuss their reasons for making the matches and, after the discussion, each student writes an essay explaining each match.

You may also vary the activity by supplying the themes and having students create their own designs based on the themes. Students can draw their designs on the chalkboard and can explain how each design expresses its theme. Or you may have the students draw their designs on the board without revealing what themes the students feel their designs reflect. The class guesses the themes and the student leads a discussion, explaining the match between the design and the theme.

## Inner Space Meets Outer Space: Shaping Metaphor

Inner space and outer space are intrinsically linked, and we are able to separate them or dramatize their union simply because we can emphasize one end of the spectrum over the other without erasing the unity. Metaphor is one of the more powerful processes behind Doorway 2. Metaphor is a playful association between items, realities, objects, subjects, and so on. Metaphor celebrates the essential unity and diversity of all things. In some way all things share a commonality, an aspect of similarity where one thing becomes the other thing in a certain way.

Metaphor is created naturally in the mimetic activity of children where anything can be anything else. A child says, "I am a tree," and for a brief moment the child has become his or her own metaphor. The child imagines him- or herself as a tree and imitates what a tree is and what a tree does. This associational play is the basis of intuition where the child gets IN-TO-IT, gets into being something else and truly understands that thing in at least a nonconscious way.

The art of creating metaphor involves imagery, free association, and language. First make two separate lists of items. Identify each item in the first list with each item in the second list: "The hammer is a car." Then use all the senses to visualize possible connections. Experiment with statements. Eliminate the statements that are untrue or weak. Following is an example of the exercise:

### The Lists

| List 1 | List 2 |
|---|---|
| Hammer | Car |
| Toothbrush | Skunk |
| Violin | Newspaper |
| Ball | Lamp |
| Foot | Tree |
| Bullets | Raindrops |

**Identification Statements**

1. The hammer is a car.
2. The toothbrush is a skunk.
3. The violin is a newspaper.
4. The ball is a lamp.
5. The foot is a tree.
6. Bullets are raindrops.

## Visualization and Experimental Statements

The hammer is a car because both are hard.
The hammer is a car because they are both driven.

## Eliminate Untrue or Weak Statements

Eliminate the first statement because it is too obvious.
The second statement has more possibility.

## An Example of Incorporating Metaphor into Writing

Like a *car* pushed to the limit at a racetrack, his *hammer* was driven down onto nail after nail at a pace so fast that the frame of the house would be finished before the quickly gathering storm shot *bullets* of frozen *raindrops* at him. Like a steady, sturdy *tree* his *foot* held to the supporting crossbeam as the final nail found its way through two beams. It was almost night and the moon like a *ball* of *lamp*light provided him enough visibility to climb down his ladder and find his way to his car. He lived close by in a rented, one-bedroom apartment. Tired and exhausted, he ate a quick supper, washed his face and hands, but looking for his *toothbrush,* which was hidden like a *skunk* in a garden of vitamins and Band-aids in a bathroom drawer, was useless. He could smell the toothpaste he hadn't rinsed from it but couldn't find the brush. He gave up.

He pulled the covers of his bed back, slid under and grabbed the paper off his nightstand. Like the fingers of a musician picking a *violin* he turned the pages of his *newspaper* while the soothing music of the newsprint faded slowly from his vision as sleep gently hugged him into the night.

While the example illustrates connections only an older student might make, the process is the same for younger students. Remember that the heart of the process is the visualization and the experimental statement.

In her extensive discussion of metaphor, Linda Verlee Williams (1983) makes an important observation: "In a highly verbal, logical style of education there is little room for mental play, yet we know that the ability to play with ideas and concepts is basic to problem solving and creativity. Metaphor allows this type of play to occur as part of the learning process, and even nonacademically oriented students respond to its appeal" (80).

## A Smorgasbord of Suggestions

The following activities have a special place behind Doorway 2. Depending on your situation, these activities have excellent, powerful potential for tapping the intuitive-imaginative domain of Doorway 2.

- Blindfolding students and having them touch and describe objects may evoke many feelings, associations, and alternative ways of describing and guessing about reality.
- Impromptu brainstorming or brainstorming out of context is a great way to generate ideas that are not restrained by logic or a particular context. For example, in the middle of a spelling test, stop students and brainstorm ideas about a story you've read or are in the middle of reading. The goal is to list as many words as possible that remind your students of the story.
- Covering captions of cartoons, having students create their own captions based on what they think is being said, and comparing their ideas to the original is a nonthreatening way for students to connect their inner and outer spaces.
- Shakti Gawain (1982) offers a great idea. She speaks of a "Creative Visualization Notebook" in which a person draws or writes about images that exhibit the philosophy "What one wants, can be." The categories are (1) affirmation (I will succeed), (2) outflow (I can give love), (3) success (I see myself succeeding in life), (4) appreciation (I appreciate flowers), (5) self-esteem (I am wonderful), (6) self-appreciation (I like how I dress), (7) healing and assistance (I will

help the old person with groceries), and (8) fantasies/creative ideas (I imagine myself floating on a cloud in a blue sky).

- Deep inner contact with nature involves a sensory experience where one stops in a forest, beach, mountain, river, or other similar place and savors the contact by concentration, familiarity, and closed-eye marination/imagining of what is taking place.
- Alton Harrison, Jr., and Diane Musial (1978) explain how the Senoi Indians share dreams in normal conversation when they wake up. Dream time is not separated from other time. Students can explore dreams for imagery and meaning. Because dreams are such a powerful source of self-understanding, they should be a natural part of the educational experience. There are nonintrusive ways a teacher can help children explore the students' dreams as content for writing, art, and the understanding of literature.
- Enjoy the sharing of things via show-and-tell at all age and ability levels. This traditional activity is not meant for just elementary school. It's a marvelous way to break through rigid safekeeping barriers kids learn to hide behind so that a bit of risk taking that is native to Doorway 2 can take place.
- Exercising that releases energy also releases ideas.
- Fantasy, directed either through inner-space visualization or outer-space art, or through simply closing one's eyes and letting go to describe an idealized world, vacation, relationship, or vocation, releases the imagination and intuitively held ideas about the self, others, and the world.
- Free association makes connections between things ordinary consciousness does not reveal. It is the basis for making metaphors.
- Foretelling the future is a form of fantasy in which you create future events, life styles, and products without being judgmental.
- Students can use gaping (staring openmouthed at anything or nothing) as an opportunity to engage in some form of reflective writing or art.
- We can hope out loud, in writing, and through art.
- Journals are ways of keeping track of intuition.
- Even if you have to orchestrate or prompt laughter, laughing before discussions or assignments will snowball into real laughter, which

releases neurochemicals that relax the body and allow for the opening of imagination.

- Mime in which students ape each other, animals, activities, or anything is excellent for stimulating precise image states.
- Mnemonic images can help students remember things. For example one might associate a hairy ape with a person named Harry to remember Harry's name. One might associate a locale or area of a room with a segment of a speech one is giving there. In the latter case the sequence of a speech is connected to areas or objects that are arranged in a left-to-right order.
- You can construct museums in classrooms at any grade level and across all ability groups and disciplines. Museums are great opportunities to display what students have learned in a classroom or a subject area over a time. When the museum is ready, students can charge other students a nickel to get in; the students who compiled the museum can act as tour guides, docents, and experts in various areas of the museum.
- Role-playing requires empathy with the intuitive/imaginative being of another person.
- Encourage students to make quick decisions, which helps students listen to their selves and their hunches and helps them feel comfortable taking risks. Students must be willing to be wrong and you must formally encourage an atmosphere in which they feel safe enough to take that risk.
- You can cultivate silent periods in your classroom so that students can listen to themselves and hear their own feelings and authentic ideas. This silence must not be perceived as a punitive consequence. Setting up silent reading days with relaxing music, pillows, and the idea of finding one's "sacred space" can go a long way toward establishing this experience.
- Telling and reading stories is a great way to begin a unit in the sciences. Joseph Bruchac and Michael J. Caduto's *Keepers of the Earth* (1988) is one of the greatest books about natural history for children. In it, the authors describe how storytelling can be integrated into science curriculum:

> Tell children a story and they listen with their whole beings. Lead children to touch and understand a grasshopper, a rock, a flower, a ray of sunlight and you begin to establish connections between children and their surroundings. Have them look at a tree—feel it, smell it, taste its sap, study its many parts and how they work. . . . Keep the children at the center of their learning encounters. Build on these experiences with activities that help them to care for, and take care of, the Earth and other people—to develop a conservation ethic. Diné (Navajo) tradition tells us that this earth is destined to be destroyed unless people live in the right way. (xxiii)

- Visualization and goal setting are powerful tools for success. Help students use the tools to work, study, work out, improve their minds and bodies, improve relationships, alleviate anxiety, and lower the risk of disease.
- Writing with denotative and connotative imagery not only improves writing but also improves reading. William P. Wharton (1985) points out that comprehension of textbook material is essentially connected to its readability, which is connected to the imagery the authors use (145–60). Denotative imagery is the description of an event as it actually happened rather than the allusion to it (as in history books). Connotative imagery is the use of symbols and metaphors to transmit ideas.

Jerome S. Bruner (1979) speaks of the relationship between intuition and the free atmosphere required to release it: "[Intuition] is founded on a kind of combinatorial playfulness that is only possible when the consequences of error are not overpowering or sinful" (102). Bruner goes on to suggest that one of the reasons so many children are turned off by math is that math teachers "proceed to teach [students] algorithms that make it seem that what [students are] doing in arithmetic has no bearing on the way in which [they] would proceed by non-rigorous means" (104). In other words, children know a great deal and have an intuitive sense of certain facts because children possess models of the world and its functions that teachers should use; children will then feel the naturalness of mathematical knowledge and procedures.

Bruner also has summed up the importance of Doorway 2: "It is important to allow [children] to use [their] natural and intuitive ways of thinking, indeed to encourage [them] to do so, and to honor [them] when [they] do well. I cannot believe that [they have] to be taught this. Instead, we should first end our habit of inhibiting intuitive thinking and then find ways of helping [children] improve at it" (105).

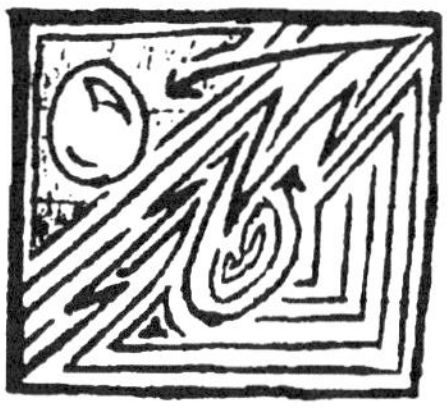

# 4. AUTOMATION

> *If we put our energies only into getting to our destination or reaching our goal, we block our sensibilities along the way. . . . When my mind gets overly bossy, I miss the perception of my senses. . . . Information from our minds can be translated instantly into activity of the body, it can also be stored, and the mind does not need to discriminate between what needs to be retained or rejected, for the body does that automatically if given the chance.*
>
> —Eloise Ristad, *A Soprano on Her Head*

## Our Bodies' Knowledge

In writing of the birth of her son, Bapu, in water, Chris Griscom (1989) states, "In truth, our body is the only one who knows exactly what is happening and at the same time can virtually alter reality at the direction of our command" (9). Later, ruminating on the moment when she had conceived Bapu, she states, "Not only do our bodies know when we conceive, but so does everyone else" (15).

Griscom avers that the body is a knower, that it possesses information, uses that information, and sends and receives it. This inherent bodily knowledge, bodily sensitivity to the environment, and bodily communication of knowledge happens automatically. I assign the concept of automation to Doorway 3.

Robert Ornstein and David Sobel (1987) underscore that the body's automatic sending and receiving of information are not, at first, within conscious awareness and control, but that they are influenced by the negatively ionized particles in the environment. The authors write of the effect of these particles.

> Air rich in negatively charged ions appears to have a refreshing and stimulating effect on us. Negative ions predominate around waterfalls, in clean mountain air, and at beaches, and disappear in polluted urban centers or enclosed spaces. The effects from minute concentrations of air ions seem to bypass the conscious part of the brain and work directly on brain chemistry and growth. Negative ions have been shown to increase brain serotonin, a neurotransmitter associated with more relaxed moods. In . . . studies, rats raised in a negatively ionized atmosphere had a cerebral cortex 9% larger than those in a nonionized atmosphere. (218–19)

An accumulation of data indicates that our bodies, like wires in an electric circuit, conduct all kinds of information into them from the outside and out of them from the inside.

Paul D. MacLean (1973) has suggested that our brains evolved in three stages, giving rise to three layers of the brain and three fundamental human behaviors (see figure 4.1). These three layers are vertically stacked within our skulls. The first layer is the reptilian, which produced territoriality and survival mechanisms such as hiding and camouflaging. The second layer is the mammalian; it ushered in behaviors such as caring and nurturing, which allowed families to survive by fulfilling inbuilt needs such as suckling and nesting. The third and most recent layer is the neomammalian, which allowed for the abstract and symbolic thought necessary for planning and survival. MacLean's basic idea is that there are three major biological-neurological potentials within human beings that account for observable behavior. When I speak of the automatic doorway I mean what MacLean terms the reptilian brain.

In commenting on the reptilian brain, Melvin Konner (1982) says, "MacLean's contribution has been to show that this structure, whether in reptiles, birds, or mammals, is not concerned with mere control of movement, but with the storage and control of 'instinctive' behavior: the fixed action patterns and innate releasing mechanisms of the ethologists" (147–48). The development of the *reticular activating system,* or the

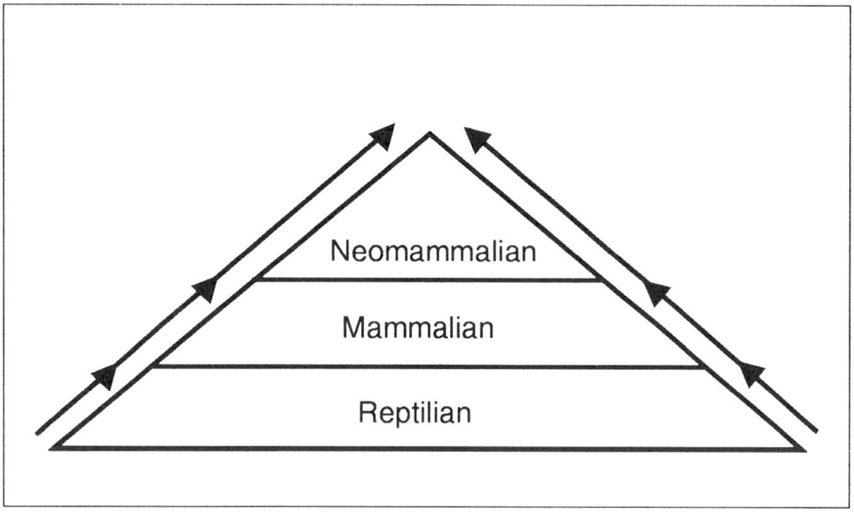


Figure 4.1. MacLean's triune concept of the brain and behavior

reptilian brain, has very much to do with programs, both physical and emotional, that are innate in their specificity. For example, smiling and crying appear to be automatic responses connected with greetings and separations. The tendency for humans to walk is automatic. Whatever external encouragement or discouragement is given either builds on or suppresses this automatic response.

The reticular activating system, a bundle of nerves stretching from the brain stem into the limbic system (medulla to the thalamus) in some way conducts stimulation in the environment into the three brains described by MacLean and creates, at first, an arousal beneath conscious awareness that is locked into both our emotional and motor systems. The body reveals its own being through clues that are muscular, chemical, and behavioral. The purpose of self-awareness is to become conscious of these psycho-physical states so that we can change the stimulus that may be causing stress, anxiety, and what Leslie Hart (1983) refers to as the "downshifting" syndrome in learning (102–11). This downshifting occurs when higher cortical function stops and the brain operates according to the survival programs of its lower structures.

We can ask some very important questions about Doorway 3. First, what does the body know that can help us make learning more compatible with its needs, rhythms, and potential for arousal and sedation? Second, what is the relationship between arousal, sedation, and learning? Third, can we point to factors in the physical and psychological environment of a classroom that affect the body either negatively or positively and condition lesser or greater learning experiences? Fourth, while the word *instinct* may be much too narrow to use in reference to human activity, is there a way around the perception that built into the lower brain are instincts that are like antennae, sending and receiving coded messages about the nature of the individual and the environment around the individual? Paying attention to this instinct, eliciting what it knows and understanding what it is saying, may be one of the ultimate skills in teaching. Honoring this instinct is important to the prebonding processes necessary for bonding and a lifelong desire to learn. Fifth, is it possible to interpret the physical data of students so that we can create Rorschach-like symbols that represent a new kind of typology, giving us immediate information about the person's intellectual, emotional, and stylistic preferences and potentials?

## An Activity to Shake Up the Locked-up Information

1. Have two students stand ten feet apart, facing each other. Ask one student to walk slowly toward the other and stop when he or she gets halfway. Ask the student who has been standing still to report whether or not he or she could feel any kind of energy or vibration from the other student.

   Next ask both students to move toward each other very, very slowly and to report any energy they feel. Then have two more students line up five feet behind the first two. Tell the first two to close their eyes. Tell the second two to move slowly, inch by inch, toward the backs of the first two. Ask the first two to raise an arm when they first sense (not hear) the energy or vibration coming from behind them. Continue this process until your whole class is involved. All your students will be standing, eyes closed, at various distances behind the first two students.
2. Instruct your students to keep their eyes closed and give each student an inflated balloon with his or her name on it. At your

signal, your students are to toss the balloons gently up and concentrate on sensing the balloons as they move through the air, touch the students' bodies, fall to the floor, and stop moving. In the silence ask students if they can sense where the balloons are. Ask each student to point to where he or she thinks his or her balloon is.

3. Next, so the students will not be alarmed, inform the class that you are going to pop a balloon several feet from each person's head and ears. Their anticipation of the balloon popping is important. Be sure to ask each student to try to feel how the whole body reacts when you pop the balloon. Ask them, "Where in your body other than your ears did you sense the balloon popping?"
4. Discuss and allow students to write about their experience. Have them exchange notes on what they felt and thought of the activity. Finally, play relaxing music in the background and ask students to write freely of the whole experience. They can go back later and refine what they write.

## The Natural Wisdom of the Body

Our culture reels under the dualism of mind and matter. The body is seen as something to be suppressed or changed (lose weight/get muscular), as the source of ever more uncontrolled passion (eros), or as the repository and channel of death (thanatos). Most of us live in a delicate, overly sensitive state of fear, denial, and oppression of the body no matter what we proclaim sexually, athletically, or dietetically. Why? Because there is a dimension of the body we almost miss: it is the contact point between two worlds, spirit and matter. In a sense the distinction between these two worlds becomes meaningless when people have certain kinds of peak experiences.

Doorway 3 is the part of the brain closest to the rest of the body and Earth itself. It is the primary conduit for both body and Earth energies, which the brain processes in order to sedate or arouse us. In general, Doorway 3 is an automatic sensor and recorder of positive and negative states of sedation and arousal within a person and outside in the social and physical environment. We use the word *automatic* to describe these processes because the body's sensory awareness is always there and is initially beyond our awareness or our control. One hears stories of Native Americans or other native peoples who know the land, the forests, the animals—nature in general. Of what did this knowledge consist? It was Doorway 3, automatic wisdom, a sensory contact with the self and the world that has become dulled in most teachers.

Why has it become dulled? Because as a culture, we have had to develop a strong denial mechanism to function within the negative social and physical forces around us. We have also denied our own deepest feelings of satisfaction and those sources of satisfaction that heal. Is it any wonder that this basic denial response reveals itself as a skepticism that is ruled by the negative arousal state called fear? As teachers we very much need to reclaim our bodies (whatever their size or shape) and begin listening to them so that we can unleash for ourselves and our students the affirmations of life for which education should be providing the tools of expression.

## Proprioception

We all have three receptors that are stimulated by and that monitor external events (basic sensations of sight, sound, smell, taste, and touch); internal events (hunger, fatigue); and events within muscles, joints, and the inner ear. It is our proprioceptors ("self feelers") that guard these latter sensations.

Proprioception monitors and adjusts our place in space, gives us balance, and shapes our bodies. As Arthur Balaskas (1979) notes, "Proprioception is our most basic sense of connection to the earth, involving the body's relationship with gravity, space and the atmosphere. While you are reading this, your eyes and thinking process are active in the foreground. Yet, in the background your proprioceptive sense is active, making you aware of your body—of its breathing, for instance, and its spatial magnitude and position" (223).

Proprioceptors relay messages back and forth between body and brain, allowing the brain-body duality to maintain the body's posture, balance, and place or extension in space, as well as the evolving structure that gives the body its shape. All of these functions occur beneath conscious awareness, and when the body begins to deteriorate, we become conscious of proprioceptive information at first through pain, stiffness, and a sense of gradually reduced capacity to move through space with ease. Ignoring this early proprioceptive information eventually results in two things: (1) adaption of the body to physical limitations and (2) loss of proprioceptive information; that is, the body becomes habituated to restricted movement, and sensory information is slowly but surely minimized. In time we lose touch with our bodies, and the sense that we are carrying around something foreign increases. We also become diseased, reflecting all that is diseased around us and all that we have denied within us.

There are few teachers who do not, in some way, experience grief and carry with them grief for the dying body they have become. Nothing deepens that grief more than the incredibly alive bodies of our students. Teachers often have a hidden agenda that has something to do with jealousy of children and teenagers and repression. This repression causes teachers to fail in addressing the proprioceptive wisdom of their bodies, which often expresses itself in a teacher's failure to understand not only the bodies of students but the fact that wisdom itself involves self-awareness, and self-awareness requires proprioceptive contact with the body.

## A Proprioceptive Activity for Children in Grades 6–12

Doctors Tobin Simon and Linda Trechter-Metcalf, founders of the Proprioceptive Writing Center of Portland, Maine, write of proprioception as an "inner intelligence" and a "secret sense." They explain that "through inner intelligence, we access our thoughts and discriminate among them; in short, know ourselves. Because inner intelligence is stimulated by the form we teach, and because we approach meaning through feeling, we call this practice 'Proprioceptive Writing.'" (*Proprioceptive Writing Center Bulletin*). In other words, there are activities that involve written expression that taps proprioceptive information.

The following activity, "Proprioceptive Writing," owes much to the work of Simon and Metcalf, who have brought to the act of writing a new depth and respect that one would have thought difficult in an age where the written word is supposed to be eclipsed by visual technology.

You may do this activity effectively with most age groups. Adapt the activity according to the time you have and the circumstances under which your students will be writing. Try to have at least one candle for every two students. Play soothing baroque music. Allow ten to fifteen minutes for the first part of the exercise and return to the exercise several days later to allow students to revise, edit, and "spiff up" their writing. This exercise takes between thirty-five and forty minutes.

1. Darken any windows, turn off the lights, and light the candles. Be sure each student has a pen or pencil and paper.
2. Tell your students that you will be playing a selection of Mozart's music and that you would like them to relax and let the glow of the candlelight and sound of the music seep into their bodies and minds. Tell them that at some point they will sense the need to write and that they should follow the need and begin to write. Also tell them that it is not the time to judge what they write but to let their feelings express themselves through the writing. Also tell them that if they choose not to write or do not feel like writing, it is okay for them not to write.
3. Play the music for several minutes, then ask the students to focus on what parts of their bodies feel the music and what parts do not feel the music, such as behind their knees or the backs of their heads. Suggest again that if they are relaxing and sensing their feelings and what their bodies have to say, they may be moved to write. Ask those who have begun to write to continue and ask those who have not begun to write to try to take advantage of the urge to write.
4. Allow up to ten minutes to elapse. At the end of ten minutes, ask students to end their writing. Ask for a minute of reflective silence.
5. Take a break.
6. Ask for volunteers to share their writing. Do not require anyone to share. When the sharing is over and students have had an opportunity to ask each other questions about their writing, request that they remain silent for a minute. Ask that the students nearest the candles blow them out.

7. Suggest that students use the process at home to finish and edit their writing.
8. Hold individual conferences with students to discuss their writing. Be sure to inquire how their bodies felt during the exercise and what their bodies were telling them about themselves.

This proprioceptive writing activity is a wonderful way to involve parents and children in an experience that allows them to listen carefully, respectfully, and openly to their own "inner intelligence" or "secret sense," where body and spirit meet to make sense of life. The exercise also helps them listen to each other more effectively.

## A Proprioceptive Activity for Children in Grades K–5

The following activity is appropriate for children at the lower elementary level. It takes into account the Doorway 3 need for ritual and mime. Children repeat events automatically until the events become rituals. The activity makes children feel secure, helps them create a sense of place all their own, and creates a sense of belonging. Children are also natural imitators and love to pretend to be various kinds of animals, objects of nature, and objects of technology. This activity draws from this automatic preconceptual drive for safety, belonging, and experimentation.

1. Ask the children to stand in an open area where they can exercise and imitate freely.
2. Play a tape of nature's sounds, such as Gordon Hempton's *Dawn Chorus: Earth Sounds,* in the background. The American Museum of Natural History has recommended this tape as a marvelous example of the sounds of nature from across America.
3. Ask the children to watch you carefully as you raise your arms parallel to the ground and make slow undulating motions with them, like an eagle in slow-motion flight. Ask the children to close their eyes and do as you are doing. Ask them to concentrate on the motion of their arms and whether or not the motion is relaxing, tiring, easy, or difficult. Then ask the children to concentrate on what parts of their arms feel

relaxed and what parts stiff and strained. See if the children can focus on the parts of their arms that feel these ways.

4. Ask the children to list the animals they would like to imitate. List the names of the children in the order in which they will imitate their animals.
5. Begin with the child first on the list. Ask that child to imitate the animal he or she chose, then ask the rest of the children to imitate him or her. Continue through your list until every child has led the imitation.
6. Ask the children to decide which animal was most difficult to imitate and which was easiest. Ask the children individually what made the imitation so difficult and see if they can point out the parts of their bodies in which they felt this difficulty.
7. Have your children do the following activities based on their responses to step 6.

   *Writing:* Students write a story with one of the following titles: "It's Easy and Difficult to Be an Animal," "The Little Boy/Girl Who Thought He/She Was a ______, ""The Day I Turned into a ______."

   *Drawing:* Students illustrate their stories, drawing their animals once from memory and once from a picture of the animal.

   *Performing:* Videotape the children as they read their written pieces, display and explain their drawings, imitate their animals, and finally explain how their bodies felt when they did the imitation.

## Computer-Assisted Energy Field Readouts

Although Doorway 3 involves the body, its focus is not so much on motion as it is on our ability to be aware of our bodies as contact points for information that is waveform, pulsating, and vibrational. Our bodies are antennae that give and receive messages coded as peaceful, relaxing, compassionate, and nonaggressive at one pole, and those coded as warlike, disturbing, cruel, and aggressive at the other pole. Other codes that are polar involve messages of life and death.

The body is the primary source of information for the brain. Indeed, the body *is* the brain, for in its cells are the genetic codes that determine a great deal about the kind of brain an individual possesses. The body knows the negative and positive poles of reality because it is aware of its own fluctuations in energy levels, feeling states, and rhythms. These are raw data that form the background of all communication, dialogue, and solitary self-awareness.

Teachers who are ignorant of the body as a source of this primary information create poorer academic and curricular programs. Every child that comes to every school is a living, pulsing data bank of information. Each child is his or her own background-coded, brain-body system that needs understanding and room for expression in order to release the higher cortical functions of the brain and to embrace the realm of symbolic understanding and communication.

For some educators, this concept will seem farfetched, but someday, all schools will offer the following: As students come through the doors of their classrooms, a device in the doors will read the energy fields of students and terminals will print out corporate profiles and anonymous individual profiles. The goal of the readout will be to help students' resensitize their bodies to the traffic of incoming and outgoing information that allows optimal learning to take place. From these readouts, teachers will get a sense of the underlying data that might help students follow or hinder them from following the day's plan. Teachers will be able to use the information to suggest ways in which the students can make the most effective use of their day. For example, one child might need to sleep during study period or to eat certain foods in the school cafeteria on a given day. The readout might suggest sounds, smells, and visuals to enhance the classroom activity. Of course, teachers could use the system to bring their own bodies back into balance so that they can be as clear, creative, and helpful to students as possible.

## The Effect of Sound upon the Body

Enough data exist to suggest that using music and natural sounds as part of "stage setting" gives students the greatest opportunity for taking in information and expressing it, especially in writing, across all subject areas. Allan Bloom (1987) comments on the relationship between music and the development of the mind. Bloom suggests that liberal education requires the use of feeling, sentiment, and passion as part of a balanced and harmonious marriage with reason. He goes on to state,

> Education is not sermonizing to children against their instincts and pleasures, but providing a natural continuity between what they feel and what they can and should be. But this is a lost art. Now we have come to exactly the opposite point. Rock music encourages passions and provides models that have no relation to any life the young people who go to universities can possibly lead, or the kinds of admiration encouraged by liberal studies. Without the cooperation of the sentiments anything other than technical education is a dead letter. (80)

However controversial may be Bloom's exposition of the decline and fall of U.S. education, as caused by both the larger culture and the policies and practices in our educational institutions, he does finger a basic problem fundamental to the brain's programmatic requirements for higher cortical processing and rational inquiry. Doorway 3 is the first contact the brain-body system has with the overall vibratory quality of the environment. The system resonates, physically echoes what is around it. When submerged in some rock music, the brain-body system can fail to become an adequate prologue, channel, or entrance into the higher brain functions of Doorways 1 and 2. The system may drown if the beat, rhythm, and pulsation are too fast, too chaotic for purposes of causal inquiry and intuitional/imaginal release.

Some rock music affects feelings, sentiments, and passions in such a way that it tends to shut down reason and imagination. Doorway 3's primary activity is arousal and sedation of the entire brain-body system. Like all systems, the brain-body seeks homeostasis, and rock music tends to maintain the system in a state of arousal too long. The system becomes so accustomed to releasing endorphins to cope with this prolonged vibrational abuse that it cannot release the endorphins under less stimulation. In other words, in time the system becomes addicted to the music, for paradoxically, the pain it sometimes creates causes the brain to release pleasure. One gets hooked, saturated, and driven by the beat, not into an altered state of consciousness or trance connection with the powers of the unconscious mind, but rather with volcanic forces of turbulent overdrive of the senses. Then there is no time or inner space for reason and imagination, whose workings depend not only on arousal but also on sedation, relaxation, and a harmonic vibration, a music that opens up reason and sets free the wild things of the imagination.

On the other hand, there are forms of rock and roll whose driving beats are based on the trance-inducing qualities of tribal music. These beats can transform awareness, expand the imagination, and launch the mind into a depth of understanding that enables it to seek form through poetry, art, story, and design. No one expresses this positive potential of rock and roll more potently than Mickey Hart and Frederic Lieberman (1991). They state that "loud music and vigorous dancing can produce a form of egolessness that is the ground for any sacred exploration" (119). Some rock-and-roll rhythms and vibrations can lock the brain into a pulsation that serves learning by giving to the brain a level of arousal that shuts out competing information and, in a sense, produces focused states analogous to those induced by deep relaxation.

What, then, is the music or the sound that harmonizes and marries sentiment, feeling, and passion with reason and intuition/imagination? Although listening is primarily an activity of the ear, it is also an activity of the whole body, especially the skin, joints, and skeletal structure. The major principle of Doorway 3 is that the body itself is the ground for higher intellectual and spiritual awareness. A major purpose of the body is to become an ever more refined conduit for energy into and out of ourselves. Don Campbell (1991) states,

> There was no doubt to ancient healers and philosophers that music is the bridge between body, soul and earth. Our vocabulary may have shifted during the past two thousand years, but the awareness of vibratory fields of energy as the life force of the body is an emerging realization in medicine. The influence of vibration on creation was acknowledged through the time of Kepler. The modern world is coming to honor these visions of perfect number systems, music of the spheres and God's mystic nature revealed through number, pattern and proportion. *An older part of the brain* is in touch with the power of these principles, and newer research suggests that they are evolutive and creative. (6; emphasis added)

In the same anthology Campbell includes his interview with ear specialist Dr. Alfred A. Tomatis. Dr. Tomatis points out that there are sounds that charge the brain and sounds that tire it. In response to the question "What sort of sounds do you use in re-charging people?" Dr. Tomatis said, "At various stages in the process I will use sounds such as a recording of one's mother's own voice, filtered to simulate the listening one has prenatally. Also, music, but not just any music, because each kind has different results. Two kinds in particular have given me results in every corner of the world: the music of Mozart, and Gregorian chant from the Abbey of Solemnes" (18). It so happens that baroque music, of which Mozart is a master, is the musical basis for Dr. Georgi Lozanov's method of accelerated learning, which is now gaining acceptance throughout the world.

Music is not a peripheral business. We must take into account the effects that sound and music have on both physical and mental development. Yet most teachers have no idea how to use music, nor have they persevered in making it an integral part of their teaching/learning philosophy and methodology.[1]

## Setting Up a Sound and Musical Classroom

Integrating sound and music in the classroom requires basic equipment: a good cassette player or, if possible, a CD player; a basic classical and new age collection (good starters are Jean Pierre Rampal's classical interpretations, the works of Ray Lynch, Pachelbel's Canon in D Minor, Enya's *Watermark,* most works by Kitaro); a basic collection of rock tapes (include your favorites); and a basic collection of natural sounds (ocean waves, rainfalls, and so on). Be sure you don't allow your students to perceive the cassette player as a chance to play their favorite tunes. They have enough opportunity for that outside your class. Designate the equipment as your own; you will use it to provide the sounds you have decided are an important part of your classroom curriculum experience. Consider using music or sounds during these times:

- when students are working in groups
- during quiet reading
- when students are writing

1. For a more detailed discussion of sound, rhythm, and music in the classroom, as well as specific musical suggestions, see *Rhythms of Learning: Creative Tools for Developing Lifelong Skills* by Don Campbell and Chris Brewer (Tucson, Ariz.: Zephyr Press, 1991).

- when students are taking tests
- periodically when you are presenting material (as long as the sound or music is comfortably in the background and not interfering with or competing with your voice for attention)
- at times of greetings and good-byes to individual classes or during transition periods if you are with one class all day
- during quiet research or project work

Does this approach work? A good way to answer this question is to share with you an essay written by a tenth-grade student whose English teacher uses sounds and music as an integral part of classroom work.

## Classical Music: A Panacea

One aspect of English class that I felt enhanced the learning environment was the classical music that was played. It was very relaxing, it helped clear my mind, and helped me focus on the task at hand.

The classical music was very relaxing. My body was able to let go of all the stress that was created in other areas of my life. Also, my worries seemed to run out through my fingertips. Relaxing is a key step to performing to my potential and beyond. During vocabulary tests I usually freeze up, especially when I only have five minutes to study the words, but with the music on, my nerves relaxed and let me go on with my work. Probably the main reason I do not do as well as expected on exams is because I let my nerves take over. With the music playing, my body just lets go and lets my imagination juices flow freely.

The music helps my mind which is essential in the learning process. If my mind is cluttered up with existential material, I would not be able to learn as much, or as fast, as I would if my mind was clear. I believe this has been proven scientifically. The music seems to wipe the slate clean and make my mind a sponge absorbing everything that comes its way. This panacea also makes me more receptive to new ideas, such as the mnemonic vocabulary, which was new to all of us this year. If the music had not been playing, and clearing my mind, maybe I wouldn't have accepted that new form of learning vocabulary.

The classical music helps me focus on the task at hand. Whether it be vocabulary or essays, I was always ready to tackle it. This is because the music allowed me to focus all of my energies on the task because I was not worrying about unimportant material. This year it seemed as though I did not do a lot of work. However, I started getting back

> projects, essays and vocabulary tests, and it was remarkable the amount of work I did. The reason I felt I did not do a lot of work was because the music took my mind off the work itself and just let me go about my business.
>
> I strongly believe the classical music made a great difference in class this year. All these topics I have discussed work together like a jigsaw puzzle to create the best atmosphere and mood in which to learn. Try to follow me on this one. The music helped me to relax, that cleared my mind which helped me to focus on the task at hand which helped my grades. Did you follow? It is okay if you didn't. All you need to understand is that the classical music was a healthful behavior that had a long, wonderful holistic effect.
>
> —S.F.

This student's essay testifies to the essence of the rationale for incorporating sound/music into the classroom: (1) it relaxes, and relaxation is an important key in learning, studying, and performing; (2) it makes a lot of work seem like no work at all; and (3) it is a natural motivator.

## Singing the Body Postured

As elementary as it may seem, the postural position of the body both influences what we receive from the environment and what we send into it. Jean Houston (1982) explains, "In the state of good posture, which is indeed a state of being, your body will feel very light, almost weightless, and will seem less dense—as if your head were a kite and the rest of your body the tail dangling lightly from it" (11).

You may read students' postures, your own posture, and other teachers' postures and comprehend the kind of immediate relationship these individuals are having with their environment, including people, places, and things. Figure 4.2 illustrates three fundamental postures: backward, balanced, and forward. The arrow indicates the direction of forward movement. (A) is a backward posture implying carefulness, shyness, and, in its pathological form, depression. (B) is a balanced posture and implies a balanced relationship with the environment, in which both self and others share in the creating of life. (C) is a forward posture that implies aggressiveness and a "getting things done" relationship with the environment. In its pathological dimension it can mean violence that stems from paranoia.

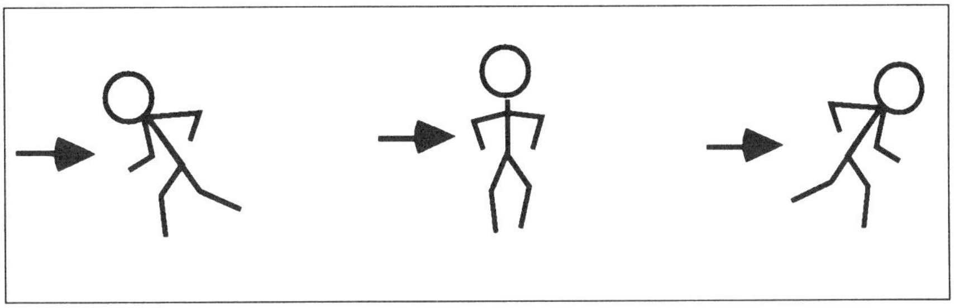

Figure 4.2. Backward, balanced, and forward postures

## Posture-Building Classroom Activity

Ask students to lie on the floor, looking straight up at the ceiling. Ask them to imagine that this posture is the one they have when they stand up. Ask them to stand up and to assume the posture they had while lying on the floor. Request often that they breathe slowly and deeply, inhaling through the nose and exhaling through the mouth. Watch the posture that each student gradually assumes and attempt to get a profile of (A), (B), and (C) postures. At some point ask students what they think their typical postures are. See if their self-perception matches the profile you constructed from your observations.

## Implications of Postural Readings for Learning

With children and teenagers, posture reveals how they were treated, what kinds of behavior they are likely to engage in, and what images they have of themselves. If any of these is negative, the negativity will take residence in their bodies and act on their postures like architects and masons who construct a building. Just as from a building you can conclude something about the person who designed it, the masons who built it, and the society that lives in and uses it, so too with the human body can you draw some likely conclusions.

An article in *Brain-Mind Bulletin* describes Stuart Heller's concepts about movement psychology, stating, "The historic personality becomes embedded in the neuromuscular layer. Like writing in concrete, this 'postural personality' reflects long-term habitual responses. Until it becomes more fluid—like writing in water—the internal movement is stopped. If the postural personality does not change, he said, a new understanding is only a change of mind, not a transformation." ("Movement Psychology Freeing 'Postural Beliefs,'" 2). In other words, what kids know and what they are or are not open to knowing is encoded in their limbs, joints, and muscles. Since education is meant to help children discover themselves, to encourage and nurture creative intelligence, and to enable both lifelong learning and informed participation in life, it is important to find out how students experience their own bodies, that primary contact point between self and world. If children and teenagers don't change, grow, and question the world around them, their rigidity (the "closed door policy" of a closed mind) will be present in the body. For Doorway 3 to serve the whole brain in all of its potential, the programmed muscular and joint memories in the body need to be replaced by a new program of movement and massage that will allow new knowledge to transform the whole child and encourage that child to continue the quest for a loving, honest, compassionate, and searching relationship with others, the natural world, and the self.

## Curricular Conclusions from Postural Readings

Some of these conclusions may seem radical, but remember that *radical* comes from the base word *root.* Not only do these curricular conclusions attempt to get at the root of things but they address the body as the root from which higher intelligence grows. The conclusions are these:

- Schools need people who understand the energy systems of the body, who know various massage and movement therapies, and who become part of an overall team approach to clusters of from one hundred to three hundred students.
- Special educators need to expand their interactions with students to include these therapies, which are necessary to remove and heal blockages of the learning process.
- Teachers and students need to repattern classroom events to include body awareness exercises so that the split between mind and body is eliminated and the body is understood as the base from which learning takes place.
- Students having a difficult time academically and behaviorally should be recorded on videotape and allowed to study the tapes

with a counselor to increase their primary awareness of their bodies and intentionally change how they carry and move their bodies.
- Teachers and students must learn acupressure techniques that take into account the holographic coding of parts of the body. (The ears, hands, and feet contain these codes for the entire body.) Such knowledge gives students a powerful tool with which to change their own body states to optimize the mind for learning.

## Construction of a Doorway 3 Reptilian World

Doorway 3 opens to a paradoxical world where primitive sensory awareness is shot through with cosmic significance; a human is never merely a stimulus/response pattern of behaviors, because time and space occur between stimulus and response. What the human being does with primitive needs built into the base brain is reform them into activities and rituals that serve both the base brain and the higher cortical centers, which together form a unified whole.

Our cultures influence how we deal with these base-brain, reptilian traits. Often we bypass, suppress, ignore, deny, or even attack them. We are still programmed by our dualisms and afraid of our bodies, alienated from the messages within them, and numbed to the enormous garden of earthly delights they may offer. We can make the rituals that celebrate body wisdom and the reptilian, base-brain contacts within the network of sensations and fields of energy part of our classrooms. As teachers we must strive to reunite body and spirit wisdoms so that they mirror each other, teach each other, and become more consciously the wholes that they never cease to be. Instead of subtly discarding body and spirit as opposites in our classroom rituals, we must nurture them holistically.

Our attempt to avoid base-brain Doorway 3 realities is like crossing a bridge over a beautiful river and not taking note of the river. Not only is the river beautiful (and terrible in the sense of its awesome power), but it contains information, sounds, reflections, visual patterns, and ripples from objects sitting in it and moving through it. If you have ever commuted to work through such beauty, such subtle information, you understand the need to ritualize this experience daily because it affects the whole day itself.

What are the rivers and streams we have avoided in our culture as we have crossed over our bridge of days as professional teachers? And what rituals do these streams and rivers suggest we begin to cofashion with our students so that the sensory information they contain feeds our psyches with awareness of "where it's at"? Morris Berman (1984) gives us a clue in his comments about a holistic society:

> Holistic society is thus coming upon us from a variety of sources that cut across the traditional left-right political axis. Feminism, ecology, ethnicity, and transcendentalism (religious renewal), which ostensibly have nothing in common politically, may be converging toward a common goal. These holistic movements do not represent a single social class, nor can they even be analyzed in such terms, for by and large they represent the repressed 'shadows' of industrial civilization. (282)

Berman goes on to list these shadows and the goals that are associated with their manifestation. The repressed shadows include the feminine, the wilderness, the child, the body, the creative mind and heart, the occult, and peoples of nonurban and regional peripheries of Europe and North America. Our goals for recovery must include recovery of our bodies, our health, our sexuality, our natural environment, our archaic traditions, our unconscious mind, our rootedness in the land, and our sense of community and connectedness to one another (Berman 1984, 282).

## K–12 Base Brain Reptilian Awareness Rituals

We can help children recover their bodies in the following ways:

- Rhythmic breathing accompanied by a daily entry in a log about how one's body feels (being specific about painful and pleasurable feelings)
- Periodic use of nap time
- Stretching
- Forming circles, using slow-motion movement, holding hands
- Miming martial arts movements, accompanied by occasional bursts of breath

- Eating healthy snacks, such as fruits and nuts, at snacktime
- Touch metaphoring: using various objects with different textured surfaces and asking children to compare themselves to the surfaces (that is, deciding which surfaces remind them of themselves)

We can help our students recover their health by offering the previous activities and those that follow:

- Having them keep journals on what they are and are not doing that is conducive to good health.
- Making a healthy breakfast available to those who, for some reason, miss it.
- Having regular small-group discussions on health issues, moderated by experts in the areas.
- Engaging in visualizations that focus on scanning the body, isolating areas of pain or discomfort, and bringing to those areas images of healing and relaxation.
- Holding regular small-group discussions on issues of abuse and neglect and their effect on health. These groups require security and trust so that participants don't feel locked into their bodies and unable to say what they need to say. You must screen students so that those with serious issues can receive counseling and therapy instead of participating in the group alone.
- Holding a once-a-month healthy meal get-together of all teachers and students and inviting a guest speaker whose talk will appeal to the kids.

Classroom activities that promote recovery of our sexuality might include the following:

- Regular small-group discussions of gender issues; having boys and girls meet separately first is necessary in grades 7 through 9 and may prove beneficial in other grades, as well.
- Development of a classroom statement on gender issues, not to exclude the connection between sexuality, love, celebration, tenderness, and compassion (to be read at least once a week at the beginning of the day).
- Having students create poetry, essays, art, and drama about gender and presenting the works to their peers.

- Male-female mirror movement exercises.
- Creation of group "families," where family roles are assigned along with character and behavioral descriptions for each role. Give each group a problem to solve as a family and within each prescribed role. Following the dramatization the class discusses how the roles and the contributions of each family member affected their gender identities and expectations.
- Once-a-month talks by guest speakers from a variety of ethnic groups whose topic is male and female roles in their cultures.
- Student presentations about important males and females in their lives, followed by questions and answers (and perhaps the recitation of the classroom statement on gender roles).

To facilitate the recovery of our natural environment, try the following:

- Maintain collections of rocks, fish, flowers, and insects along with a changing series of posters that pay homage to our natural environment. Each day a student selects some element of the collection to celebrate by writing a piece that identifies him or her with the object, for example, "I celebrate myself, for I am a mountain."
- Create, use, and maintain a classroom recycling center.
- Go on brief daily walks to a preselected natural spot, gather in a circle, and give thanks to the wonder by addressing it as brother or sister, the natural world ("brother sun, sister moon").
- Have a moment of silence in which you visualize the interconnection of all things. You can start with the fact that the feet are connected to the floor of the classroom, the floor is connected to the building, the building is connected to the ground, the ground stretches for miles and is connected to the forest and the seashore, the forest is connected to the animals that live in it, and the seashore is connected to the sea, which is connected to the creatures that live there, and so on.
- Place a natural object in the middle of the room. Beside it place a shoe box. Have students write a brief note to the object, and with great care walk one by one to the object, place the note in the box, and respectfully and affectionately touch the object.

- Maintain a permanent bulletin board dedicated to the natural environment and distribute the responsibility for maintaining it among the students. Each day give the class a few minutes to organize themselves for the purpose of maintaining it.
- Assign to each student an animal, a vegetable, and a mineral or other natural resource to learn about. Once a week gather in a circle to share information and answer questions about what the students have learned.

Classroom activities to promote recovery of our archaic traditions might include the following:

- Periodically honor the wisdom that comes with age by inviting an older person to the classroom for a question-and-answer period focused on that person's time of youth and on advice the person might give to children growing up in the world today.
- Have students choose a traditional craft (stained glass, weaving, calligraphy, metalworking) to which they rhythmically return and, with relaxation music and sounds in the background, work quietly and attentively until they complete it.
- Find out if there are any dowsers among the students. Periodically take all the students on a dowsing walk after they have created their own dowsing tools.
- Familiarize students with the power and meaning of gems. Tell them about the signatures left on smaller realities by larger ones (for example, the palmist's belief that the soul signs itself on the palms of our hands or the astrologer's belief that the stars, sun, planets, and moon influence our lives).
- Have students make masks that represent their connection to the elements: earth, air, fire, and water. Have them create a fifth "alchemical mask" that combines all these forces. Students then choose the mask that represents how their own bodies feel, don the mask, gather in a circle, and express why they are wearing that mask that day.
- Forecast weather for various parts of the world after silently visualizing a geographical spot and focusing on the effect the weather has on one's body. Check the accuracy of the forecast each time you do this activity and keep a log.

- Conduct extrasensory perception experiments with a deck of playing cards. Each child is given one card face down. Each person closes his or her eyes, places one hand on the card, and tries to guess what the card is. Keep a record of the guesses and the actual cards.

To help students recover their unconscious minds, try the following:

- Create or find abstract designs or visuals that have no literal meaning. Pass out the designs to your students and have them write about the designs. Finally, ask the question, "How does your body feel when you look at the design?"
- After discussions on dreams, ask students to begin keeping a dream journal. After several weeks, share excerpts from the journals. On days when students cannot remember a dream, they can make up a dream and place a check next to the description to distinguish the description from actual dreams.
- Have students develop collections of natural objects (feathers, rocks, pieces of wood, and so on) whose feel and presence is special to them. Make the collection a regular part of show and tell.
- Set up a classroom museum of paintings, natural elements, natural snacks, and various classical pieces of music. Provide candlelight as the only light. Do not allow talking for one-half hour and instruct students to keep journals of their thoughts during the half hour. Afterward, have a time to share, then ask students to choose something from their journals as the basis for a longer piece of writing and some form of visual/artistic expression.
- Ask children to imagine fog at night with a single light appearing in the distance. Ask them to make a list of things that the light could be. After having students share their responses, ask students to select one explanation that might represent something about themselves. Ask them to write about it.
- An activity that often works well with students who exhibit behavior problems is to show movies that focus on animals, such as one of the National Geographic specials. Tell students that animals often have traits similar to humans' traits and that you want the students to think about traits they identify with during the movie. Discuss the movie afterward and then have the students write about how the animals reminded them of themselves. Next, have students

draw pictures of the animals, placing their heads on the animals' bodies. To conclude, have students write brief essays; the titles should combine students' first names with those of the animals.
- Periodically give each student a clear copy of a face of a person that the student does not know. After students have had time to study the faces quietly, have them write paragraphs about the face they chose. Have them focus on the following: How do I feel as I look at this face? Is the person a quiet or outgoing type? Is this person living or dead? When students finish, give them a few silent moments to think about the face to see if a final thought about the person comes to mind. If so, they should write it down. Then have students compare notes. Lastly, reveal who the person is along with biographical detail.

To assist the recovery of our rootedness in the land, try the following activities:

- Build a small sitting/meditation platform in the middle of a school garden, field, or forest. Use it as a quiet space where students go to sit silently and appreciate the landscape and possibly to draw sustenance for a journal.
- Allow students to "lay claim" to their "sacred space" of land around the school by staking it with their names. Use the spaces, when the weather permits, as quiet study spots for the whole class.
- In a large school garden, assign each class a section. Have your classes routinely use their garden space to build the soil, sow seeds and plant seedlings, nurture the plants, harvest, and use the harvest.
- When the weather is warm, gather with students in an open field. Have students lie on their backs, forming a circle, feet facing toward the center of the circle. Next, have them focus on the feeling of the Earth against the backs of their bodies. Then have them listen carefully (alternating ears) to the Earth. At first students may feel nothing. With patience they will sense something during both parts of the exercise.
- Again in an open field, have students stand straight and visualize themselves individually as trees, with their feet a root system that extends into the ground. Ask the following questions: What do

your roots feel like? Do your roots go through or around rocks? Can you feel underground creatures such as ants, grubs, worms, and rodents as they work their way through the soil?

- Raise money to support a local, national, or international conservation organization. Make ecological sensitivity a political reality by maintaining a letter-writing campaign to various political and business leaders in the community inviting them to visit your school to converse on ecological matters. Such letter writing might evolve into a yearly program of guest speakers with whom the school will discuss not only the environment in general but also what the visiting speakers are doing to advance the cause.

We must also recover our sense of community and connectedness to one another. The following activities are appropriate to help students do so:

- Gather in a circle and hold hands for a minute. Begin a hand squeeze that students pass around the circle. Follow this activity by affirming each other or reading briefly.
- Have students hum in unison, getting louder or softer depending on how far apart or how close you bring your forefingers. Practice until perfect and praise the whole class for having accomplished something as a group of interdependent individuals.
- Have the class develop its own sign language for such statements as "I love you," "I will help you," "We are a family," and other such communal assertions. Pick regular times when half the class signs to the other half and the other half signs back.
- Plan a party each month at which five classmates are honored and given gifts. All the students, including the five, plan and provide what is necessary for the party to be a success.
- Make some form of public service an integral part of the curriculum.
- Every other week, set aside an hour to study and celebrate a culture, tribe, or ethnic group from somewhere in the world. A good way to begin is by finding out what cultures, tribes, and ethnic groups the students come from.
- Do a "Connectedness to All Things" circle. Gather four elements (flowers or soil for earth, air for air, a lighted candle for fire, and a

bowl of water for water). Have one animal present. Gather important artifacts from cultures representing the seven continents. Include symbols of the moon, planets, sun, and cosmos. Gather in a circle with all that has been collected and find an appropriate reading that celebrates this micro- and macrocosmic interconnection we have with all things. Lastly, try the metaphor identification exercise in which each student says, "I am (something from the collection) because . . . "

While you are doing these activities, you might keep two things in mind. First, there are some activities that may seem unrealistic for inner-city or blackboard jungle schools. Yet, it is possible to create inner-city gardens and sacred spaces if you have the will to do so and if you can establish a sense of community and a personal power base. Second, while all the activities in this chapter could easily be listed as activities behind the other doorways, their purpose serves the fundamental processing mode of the base brain: the deep physical connection beneath verbal and even awareness of the positive and negative forces, energies, and vibrations that precede, permeate, and follow our consciousness of all things. Education is best when it addresses this most basic need, the reticular, reptilian-brain need for ritual, safety, security, and territoriality that is nonthreatening, positive, and nurturing.

# 5. RELATION

> *It is one of the turning points in analysis when the narcissistically disturbed patient comes to the emotional insight that all the love he has captured with so much effort and self-denial was not meant for him as he really was, that the admiration for his beauty and achievement was aimed at this beauty and these achievements and not at the child himself.*
>
> —Alice Miller,
> *The Drama of the Gifted Child*

If someone placed the following quotation before you, would you recognize from what great literary work it comes? The quote appears at the end of a novel. The main character, whose life has been torturous and whose closest ally has been murdered, speaks: "Once my fancy was soothed with dreams of virtue, of fame and of enjoyment. Once I falsely hoped to meet with beings who, pardoning my outward form, would love me for the excellent qualities which I was capable of unfolding. I was nourished with high thoughts of honor and devotion. But now crime has degraded me beneath the meanest individual" (Shelley 1965, 190).

You might have guessed that Mary Shelley's Frankenstein is speaking. In this excerpt from the monologue that ends the novel, Frankenstein, the hideous creation of science gone awry, bemoans that his need and desire for love, affection, recognition, and companionship have been thwarted by society's rejection of him, which is based on his appearance. Shelley's closing image of Frankenstein is of his retreat into total isolation upon a raft of ice, "borne away by the waves and lost in darkness and distance" (192).

Who among us has not come face to face with the Frankenstein in ourselves, our students, our colleagues, or the system in which we teach? Like Frankenstein's, our needs for love, affection, recognition, and companionship are important from the moment of our conception to the very last breath we take. If these needs are not met, all other cognitive processes are paralyzed and our personalities, thought patterns, and behavior echo the desperation of Frankenstein.

Doorway 4, relation, focuses on the right limbic, mammalian brain system, which not only processes our relationship experiences but also acts as an important gateway to memory and the higher-order thinking of the neocortex and the frontal brain. In fact, until our schools take Doorway 4 seriously, there can be no valuable lifelong learning; what we now call excellence is actually our suppression of Doorway 4.

Within Doorway 4 we deal with the feelings and behaviors that arise in the context of relationships. Love, hate, happiness, sadness, peace, anger, attraction, repulsion, bonding, alienation, sexuality, friendship, and self-worth all move about like creatures in the neurochemical ocean of the limbic brain. We know, however, that this energy cannot be divorced from what we traditionally have labeled cognition. The divorce of feeling from thinking does not have its basis in the brain.

For many, learning has been based on the idea that knowledge is primarily a noncontextual awareness of the self as thinker. From this foundation the self develops abstract formulas, theories, idioms, and propositions regardless of any sensory data, for after all, sensory data are fleeting, dependent on the fickle apparatus of the senses, and often illusory. Those with an eye toward philosophical history will recognize this as the Cartesian point of view. Recent brain research, however, shows the Cartesian model to be a naive perspective.

Psychiatrist William Gray and systems scientist Paul La Violette have conducted much research on the importance of relationships to learning. According to them "the brain uses feelings to structure information" (*Brain-Mind Bulletin* 15-2). What does Gray and La Violette's information tell us? For one thing, what we have called thoughts or abstract ideas are intrinsically permeated with an affective message. This affective message is the basis for the way we use, store, and deal with an idea itself. "When we are cut off from our feeling tones, mental connections become difficult. That is why abstract information is so hard to recall; it has no grounding in the emotionally nuanced records" (*Brain-Mind Bulletin* 15-2). To "get in touch with one's feelings" is also to create the basis for higher cortical abstract reasoning and to provide the associational cues necessary for memory. For educators the implications of Gray and Violette's work are enormous. Doorway 4 opens and closes the learning process itself.

## Gender

Assertions about gender are always uttered on shaky and shifting ground. It is dangerous to polarize male-female. It is better to suggest that there are differences that may be culture based and biased rather than to overstate the biological differences that are too often used to rationalize cultural equality. It is in this spirit that I explore gender.

Of all the characteristics a human being possesses, perhaps the one that most codes and affectively structures experience is sexual type. From the moment of conception and the announcement of a forthcoming birth, families toss back and forth fantasies about the gender of the child and the possible names to be given the child; deeper than this, parents fantasize about the roles they will play depending on whether their child is a boy or a girl. More often than not these roles are idealizations that do not represent the parents' own experiences as children but rather reflect their fantasies of what a parent ought to be.

Meanwhile, nature is already cutting the cards and dealing its gender-specific hand. We know that the potentials of boys and girls differ at birth in the following important ways:

| GIRLS | BOYS |
|---|---|
| 1. More sensitive to sound and touch | 1. More sensitive to sight |
| 2. More sensitive to faces | 2. More sensitive to objects |
| 3. More small muscle control | 3. More large muscle control |
| 4. More likely to use whole-brain thinking processes | 4. More neurally lateralized/ specialized |
| 5. Matures physically more quickly | 5. Less physically mature |
| 6. More verbally skilled[a] | 6. More skilled in higher mathematics[b] |
| 7. More prone to depression and phobias[c] | 7. More prone to heart disease, autism, dyslexia, stuttering, and schizophrenia[c] |
| 8. Live longer | 8. Die earlier |

a. Recent research indicates that males tend to have different verbal skills from females and that females mature more quickly in this area; failure to recognize these differences has led to the misplacement of many kindergarten and first-grade boys in special education classes.
b. Some recent research bears this conclusion out; however, other research suggests that boys appear to do better in these areas because the tests that evaluate the skills are gender biased.
c. Recent research has indicated that those in the counseling profession tend to diagnose women with depression, neuroses, and phobias and men with psychoses and schizophrenia even when they exhibit the same symptoms; in other words, the pronation to mental illnesses of this nature are probably not gender-based but based on the preconceived notions of men and women that psychiatrists and other counselors seem to hold.

What implications do these built-in, brain-based biases have for behavior, and what must teachers do with curricula to address these tendencies and the way the tendencies emotionally influence the learning process?

## Masculinity

For boys, experience is more "thingified." A male baby responds more readily to things than to faces when they appear in his field of vision. Also, the localization of verbal processing in the left hemisphere and the right hemisphere's lower involvement in language development make the male less able to identify language with emotion and to use language as a negotiating skill. Empowered by gross motor development, the male tends to see the world as the stage where physical contact and dramatic maxi-movements (running, jumping, kicking, wrestling) define who he is and what makes him feel good. When these tropisms are combined with cultures that are still machoarchal (chest-beating patriarchy), boys can become emotionally underdeveloped, and their feelings can cause them to mislabel or reject what "masculinity" tells them is inappropriate—holistic masculine concepts, behaviors, and learning processes—because the concepts don't "feel right." So important is this "feel right" coding of information and behavior that boys inevitably fall into some form of bonding that includes ritualized joking, sarcasm, and behavior that either reduces females to objects or implicitly denies females access to equal footing in areas of competition, leadership, or social relations.

Teachers play a key role in the development of the conceptual understanding of gender. Teachers who are observant, first of their own gender histories and then of their students' gender issues, can see these tendencies among their male students. Teachers can be crucial to either cementing or reshaping what boys learn. We can make more holistic information feel right and in doing so change how boys feel about themselves, how they feel about females, and how they feel about learning. It is important that we teach information derived from biology, neurology, and history to boys so that they can be freed from debilitating myths such as "men must be strong." Robert Gilman (1987) points to five areas through which males can begin a process that will benefit themselves, others, and the planet as a whole. These areas are understanding, modeling, training, affirmation, and transcendence.

We know that males learn how to be males from other males. Boys need to see men who have not been corrupted by the machoarchy but have attained what we might call virtues of the masculine hero. Sam Keen (1991) outlines what these virtues are in the new male hero: wonder, empathy, heartful mind, moral outrage, right livelihood, enjoyment, friendship, communion, husbanding, and wildness. Males will relearn, refeel what masculinity is through exposure to male educators who possess these heroic virtues. In addition, boys need to see these virtues in the heroes of the literature that they consume. They need to encounter such heroic themes in books, movies, discussions, writing assignments, and projects.

Classrooms should become training grounds where males deal with their feelings by using whole-brain forms of expression. Guided visualizations, dance and movement interpretation, and sound call forth these feelings and help give males a new voice, one that will help them begin or continue to develop heroic virtue. Such training in the schools should also inspire males to move toward more cooperative and caring concerns and less toward competitive separation of the self for the sake of recognition.

Masculinity is a positive trait, and it deserves activities, discussions, and assignments that serve as confirmation of the inherent goodness of maleness. Affirming masculinity does not require destroying people, places, and things in order to create a false self and an irresponsible social and planetary ego. In addition to affirming the basic goodness of masculinity, we must also affirm that each individual boy is a unique expression of his own maleness, that there are as many kinds of males as there are individuals. The last affirmation is that males know they have arrived into their maleness, that their rite of passage into their masculinity has brought them to the place where they can enjoy being male.

The final requirement in the changing pattern of masculine identity according to Gilman is transcendence. Males identify with life itself, with the cosmic source of who they are. Through this sense of connection beyond the sometimes narrow concerns of the biological family, males become conservators and protectors of all life.

### *A Classroom Activity to Celebrate Masculinity*

The following activity works best in grades 7 through 12. A perceptive teacher might study this activity and extrapolate from it a similar activity for lower grades.

Materials

A stack of magazines from which students will cut out pictures
Three-foot-square pieces of white paper
Glue, tape, crayons, and, if possible, finger paints
One cassette recorder for each group, if possible

1. Divide the class according to gender into groups of two or three.
2. Have each group create a collage filling one sheet of paper with images of masculinity that they see around them.
3. Give the groups Keen's (1991) list of masculine heroic virtues on pages 120–21
4. Discuss these heroic virtues. Then have your students create collages that reflect these masculine characteristics.
5. Have each group write and record a detailed description of both collages.
6. Each group will then select a location to hang their collages and to place their audiotapes.
7. The class will move by groups from presentation to presentation, taking notes on what they see, hear, and think about.
8. Discuss with your class the differences and similarities between the collages of each group, especially those created by females and those created by males.
9. Assign one or more of the following activities or allow your students to choose one. These activities will incorporate the information, feelings, and discussions of steps 1 through 8.

    - Write a short story with a male central character who possesses the qualities of masculinity that the student feels are important.
    - Write a free verse or rhymed poem celebrating the masculine.
    - Write an essay on masculinity.
    - Develop a short dramatic piece with a group and present it to the class.
    - Keep a journal for a specified time; in your journal reflect upon one or more of the masculine heroic virtues.

## Masculine Heroic Virtues

- *Wonder:* Males can be awestruck, appreciative, thankful, and amazed at the endless variety of life in nature and in the incredible achievements of artists, sculptors, scientists, and poets.
- *Empathy:* Males can recognize the joys and sufferings of others as if those sufferings were the males' own and can stand by those who are suffering to support them, seeing the sufferers as equals.
- *Heartful mind:* Males can use silence, solitude, recollection, and thinking about their own life histories to discover their true selves, their natural feelings, their natural thoughts. They can find themselves apart from popular culture, which struggles to define us and what we need to be happy. When they find their heartful minds they find spiritual courage, they become spiritual warriors protective of people, the land, and themselves.
- *Moral outrage:* Males can refuse to allow the powerless and the weak to be abused by society, its structures, and its individuals. They can decide to struggle against poverty, injustice, pollution, and prejudice. They can choose the role of spiritual warriors without adopting a holier-than-thou attitude.
- *Right livelihood:* Dignity, honor, and compassion can be the foundation of males' vocations, work, and daily profession. What males do for a living does not have to crush their hearts or their sense of caring for others and the world.
- *Enjoyment:* Males can develop the ability to celebrate the pleasures and delights of life and to revel in the sensuality, the silence, and the sacredness of life, because it is only through this appreciation that they can truly empathize with those who are suffering.

### Masculine Heroic Virtues (continued)

- *Friendship:* Males can share with male friends those feelings, stories, struggles, and ideas that only other males can understand; by doing so, they give and receive an acceptance and validation of their shared masculine selves.
- *Communion:* Males can overcome the isolation and competitive individualism that creates loneliness by forming communities of men whose bond is "not sports, war, business, woman bashing, drinking, [or] hunting" (Keen 1991, 177). They can realize that brotherhood and fraternity are the only ways to address the violent and destructive issues created by masculine power.
- *Husbanding:* Males can practice the care and nurturance of the places where they live. They can develop the art of inhabiting our cities, towns, and rural lands responsibly so that they protect those places from pollution and help to make them spaces where people can live freely, humanely, and healthily.
- *Wildness:* Males can maintain a relationship with the raw wilderness both in its terrain and its animals. They can give up their control over things and discover their places in the natural order of the world.

## Femininity

For girls, experience is more "personified." A female baby's response to faces is more intense than is her response to things when they appear in her field of vision. Females build upon this face-responsive tropism and respond emotionally to what they perceive in faces. Because they process language more holistically than males, their words and the stories they prefer to read reflect the emotional content of experience more. Girls' verbal skills are accentuated by control in writing (manipulation of pencils) and reading (eye movement). These skills, females' responsiveness to emotive content, and earlier physical maturing places females in the center of personal relationships and interpersonal feelings. They define their self-worth based on these personal relationships and feelings.

Very young girls have a greater awareness of their feelings and respond to tones of voice and the sense of touch more readily than boys. Their relationships with each other are built on inflections in speech and physical contact and proximity. They are more naturally intimate and communicate their feelings more easily as part of their relationships with each other. Unfortunately, this innate tendency toward intimacy, connection, and female bonding is sorely tested when girls reach early adolescence.

According to Carol Gilligan (1983), when girls reach adolescence (about twelve years old), they are faced with an unfair dilemma. Their skills and tendencies toward intimacy have become engraved in their behavior patterns, but cultural norms determined primarily by the male paradigm require that they compete with one another and stop expressing their emotional needs. Besides the message itself being somewhat contradictory, it is at odds with the intimacy patterns girls have established to that point. Suddenly girls are asked (1) to forget their needs, patterns of intimacy, and the shared habit of telling the truth, which is basic to female bonding; (2) to quit speaking out and rocking the boat, something girls up to that point are free to do partly because they express themselves from the open, honest base of intimacy they create and search for; and (3) to begin competing with each other in order to establish their autonomous and competitively derived place in society (5–23).

It is no wonder that these conflicts toss early adolescent girls into crisis after crisis, play havoc with their self-esteem, and push them into various coping mechanisms such as eating disorders, seductive behavior, and lying. It is those girls who maintain the outspoken quality they are asked to give up who set the stage for healthier and more productive years as adults. They realize that they do not have to abandon connectivity, nurturance, and care in order to achieve autonomy. They are lucky not to fall into the either/or trap that much of our unevolved society has set for them.

*A Classroom Activity to Celebrate Femininity*

You can modify the following activity according to grade level, the attention span of your students, and other characteristics of your class. In general, the activity is useful for students in elementary school through adult courses.

Materials

Art supplies, composition paper, pens, pencils, and mirrors

1. Hand out the list of affirmations of the feminine on page 124.
2. After you ask the class to study these affirmations, ask for one female and one male to read them aloud to the class.
3. This step requires an atmosphere of cooperative silence. Ideally, each person will have a mirror. Otherwise, you will have to ask students to imagine the mirrors. Ask students to look into their real or visualized mirrors. If quiet, relaxing music is available, play it softly in the background. Ask the students to think of their mirrors as magical sources of information with which they communicate telepathically. Have students ask the mirror what it means to be feminine. As they listen to the "voice of the mirror" they should write freely of what they hear. Give students about five minutes to do so.
4. Share and discuss what was written during step 3.
5. Before doing this step you might want to become familiar with poster art or invite an artist in to talk about possible ways to create posters. The time, care, and emotion students put into their posters is essential to the process. Distribute art paper and

## Affirmations of the Feminine

- To be feminine is to be.
- To be feminine is to be important, valuable, capable, and indispensable.
- To be feminine is to be intimate, nurturing, caregiving, and connected.
- To be feminine is to be an outspoken, achieving, and unique self.
- To be feminine is to be equal to the masculine.
- To be feminine is to be treated with the same high expectations and attention given the masculine in classrooms across the world.
- To be feminine is to be a person, not an object.
- To be feminine is to be.

crayons. Have each student create a poster with a feminine theme that starts with the words, "To be feminine is to be . . . "

6. Display the posters.
7. As with the activity to celebrate the masculine, the final step involves a written piece. Have each student choose one or more of the following activities:

    - Write a story with a female central character who embodies the virtues inherent in the affirmations.
    - Write a poem celebrating the feminine.
    - Write an essay analyzing the role of femininity in our culture.
    - Write a script for a short dramatic presentation.

*An Activity by which to Discover Gender Models*

This activity for understanding gender identity is intended to help students discover what they think of masculinity and femininity by having them focus on models they admire or that have played important roles in their lives. Again, my concern with the relationship of gender development to learning is this: Gender awareness is a major factor in emotional life and a central contributor to an individual's feeling state. This feeling state codes what we have traditionally labeled cognition. This state can advance or retard learning, for it is like an ocean in which information travels, and like fish in a polluted sea, information will die before it reaches its destination of the higher cortical areas of the brain if this feeling state pollutes the brain with misconceptions about gender identity.

1. Have each student brainstorm a list of males and females who have influenced him or her. The list should include family members, friends, entertainers, athletes, and any others. Have students make the lists as extensive as possible; students will be dealing with many images and reasons connected with the selections.
2. Each student selects three to five names from each list. Encourage students to conduct research on each person. They gather and take notes about each, including, if possible, pictures.

3. Each student creates two posters on 1-1/2-ft-x-2-ft poster board, one for males and one for females, then divides each poster into columns, one for each person selected. The student writes the names of the people in large letters at the top of each column, then does the following activities under the names in descending order down the columns:

    - places either a picture or a representation of the person
    - writes a fifty- to one-hundred-word biography of the person
    - draws a design that represents the person
    - writes a fifty- to one-hundred-word paragraph or essay explaining why she or he selected this person
    - lists five words, preferably nouns, that represent the qualities that make the person important

    Students should be sure the finished product is neat and cared for.

4. Display the posters.
5. Ask students to study the posters and to take notes as they move from one person's posters to another's. In addition, each student will write at least two questions about the displays that she or he will ask during step 6.
6. Meet in a large group to discuss the posters. Be sure that each student asks at least one question. The question should be addressed to the student whose posters gave rise to the inquiry. At the end of the discussion ask for volunteers to summarize what the class has learned about the models they and their classmates chose.

## Self-Esteem

An equally important influence on the feelings that advance or retard cognitive processes is our self-esteem. Clare LaMeres (1990) defines self-esteem by saying it is "how I value the labels I give myself or accept from others" (39). She explains that a positive self-image depends on what we believe to be true about ourselves: "What we believe about ourselves and our world actually creates our world, even if the belief is totally false" (44). LaMeres gives the example of a fully grown elephant that can be kept in place by a chain connected to a six-inch stake in the ground. Although the elephant could easily uproot the stake, it does not do so because when the elephant was young the chain around its ankle was attached to a tree, and when the animal attempted to escape, its ankle was hurt. Having experienced this pain when young, the elephant continues to believe that its ankle will be hurt should it try to escape, even though in reality the stake would offer no resistance should the elephant decide to get away.

Gloria Steinem (1992) reviews the enormous impact schools have had on the self-esteem of females, minorities, and in the long run on all children. She asks about students: "Do they have teachers who treat them as unique unfolding mysteries—or as people who must constantly 'measure up'?" (130) After citing studies that show a dramatic decline in students' self-esteem starting in elementary and continuing through high school, Steinem states that there is "an unusual amount of agreement on their conclusions: schools cause self-esteem to plunge for almost everyone" (130). But Steinem also believes that what we have done can be undone. "One thing is clear: the human mind can imagine both how to break self-esteem and how to nurture it—and imagining anything is the first step toward creating it. Believing in a true self is what allows a true self to be born" (157).

One of the most important goals that arises from the 7 Doorways model is that schools must, first and foremost, nurture and believe in the true selves of all who are present there: students and teachers. Our students come to us with various positive and negative feelings, images and concepts about themselves. In a similar manner teachers enter the human equation called the classroom. No one in this equation does not want to value and believe in her- or himself and maintain a positive self-image. Yet the feelings we have about ourselves often interfere with the process of learning. Like the elephant, we sometimes bring memories and images of limited and negative selves into the learning process and, through these destructive recollections, fail to grow, fail to move away from what are essentially lies. We stay tethered to a short stake that, at least implicitly, limits our range of knowledge, growth, and development.

As teachers we need to understand the "feeling forces" at work in our students, since we cannot take for granted the forces are positive. The relationship students have with themselves qualifies the relationships they have with a teacher and with the value they place on learning. The relationship a teacher has with her- or himself influences not only the way she or he teaches but also the capacity to balance empathy and challenge in the classroom each day.

The relationship between self-esteem and learning is reciprocal: learning is affected by self-esteem and self-esteem is affected by learning. For the teacher, therefore, the challenge is twofold: address issues of self-esteem to enhance the learning process and address the learning process to enhance self-esteem. Success in the classroom builds self-esteem, but the success must be real, not contrived, not watered down; it must come from our belief that our students are capable of meeting challenges. If we underestimate our students and do not challenge them enough for fear that they will not succeed, we send them a secretly coded message that we expect less of them. When students become aware of such attitudes in us, all our efforts to build success have quite the opposite effect.

The attempt to provide an environment conducive to building students' self-esteem should not become a mechanism of denial of negative attributes within our psyches. If we are naive in dealing with the self-esteem limbic issue behind Doorway 4, we will only defeat the purpose and goal of developing true self-worth. Shelly Kessler (1991) addresses this issue. Kessler focuses on recognition of the dark side, Carl Jung's "shadow" component in the human psyche. Kessler explains that at the Crossroads School the building of trust between teacher and student involves facing attitudes such as envy, greed, hatred, prejudice, sadness, depression, and lust. In referring to the Crossroads School curriculum, Kessler says, "The Mysteries program acknowledges the presence of the shadow in human nature and finds ways to deal with it directly and consciously, embracing and containing without denying or repressing it" (12).

Kessler points out that the Crossroads School has taken a path that is different from that taken by some people in the field of self-esteem. "We have parted ways with many writers, thinkers, and educators in the New Age movement, and with some in the self-esteem movement, whose programs are based on denying the shadow through positive thinking" (12). Kessler asserts the importance for teachers to be skilled at dealing with the negative in themselves and their students. She states, "A teacher who is afraid of the shadow, in him or herself and in students, cannot really open his or her heart, cannot really afford to love. Learning how to work with the shadow in oneself and in the classroom is a central challenge for a teacher seeking full presence" (12).

What is refreshing about Kessler's perspective is the sense that a teacher is free to have this mixture of darkness and light and that his or her students are similarly free. The success or failure to develop a classroom that nurtures self-esteem may depend on the way the shadow self is dealt with. Sometimes the shadow itself contains the seeds of creativity, success, and self-worth. There are times when all we need to do is help students tame it, befriend it, and let its constructive energy loose.

## An Activity for Shaking Hands with the Shadow

The following activity may be used in many ways across the curriculum to build self-esteem. The activity involves listening, writing, drawing, and discussion.

1. Read the story on pages 130–32 to your students.
2. After you read the story, divide the class into groups of three or four. Give each group one copy of the story. Ask each group to create fifteen to twenty questions about the story and to decide which five are the most important.
3. Allow about five minutes or so for each group to tackle the following question: "Did the story in any way deal with the way people see themselves, handle their problems, and deal with issues of self-image, self-esteem, and self-worth?"
4. Give groups the opportunity to change, rearrange, delete, or add to their list of questions based on the discussion in step 3.
5. Have each group select two of their top five questions to ask the whole class. Members of other groups get first crack at answering them.
6. Have each group select a member to represent it in a round-table discussion about the question raised in step 3. The rest of the class takes notes and copies down questions it will raise when the round-table participants finish.

## *The Darkness Removers*

Imagine there is a dark cloud that blocks the sun wherever it goes. If the wind blows the cloud over your house, the sun almost seems to disappear. If you leave your home, a piece of the cloud falls from the sky and enters you when you breathe in. Your body feels heavy and your eyes darken and no smile wants to visit your face. After a time the cloud leaves when you exhale, but you don't know beforehand when it might leave.

For the rest of the year the cloud plays tag with you. Dropping from the sky like a dirty marshmallow balloon, it hurtles toward you, touches your head, and disappears back into the larger dark cloud from which it came. On the day the dark cloud leaves your town, you feel warm, glowing, alive again. The sun shines and the blue sky seems especially deep and rich and vibrant. A smile returns to your face and life seems better, much better. The dark cloud moves away like a black car that has parked too long in the sky waiting to be towed away.

On the days that follow, you become aware that the dark cloud has not completely disappeared. In the brightness of the sun you notice, really notice, how all things cast a shadow. You cast a shadow that touches your feet and gets bigger or smaller as the sun sweeps across the sky.

You know that in every town there are people whose job it is to remove shadows by shining powerful lights on every shadow until the sun goes down and all shadows disappear. Eventually, in some towns the sun always shines but there are never any shadows. Life is sunny and bright all the time. But, just when everything seems perfect, the sky darkens, the sun almost disappears, and the same old dark cloud returns to those towns.

The shadow removers finally decide they will remove the dark cloud. They make a giant vacuum cleaner that pulls the dark cloud out of the sky. They trap it in a giant vacuum cleaner bag. The sun shines once again and the people return to their real job, shadow removal. All is peaceful, for throughout the town there are no shadows and never a dark cloud to block the sun. Yet, the unexpected happens.

Not long after the glow of happy days arrives, the people begin to feel irritable, angry, sad, and dreary. It is as if the dark clouds and shadows, having no place to go, show up inside everyone. Though this can't be true, it feels this way to everybody.

However, all is not lost. Those who have the job of shadow and dark cloud removal also take on a third job, remover of all bad, dark feelings inside. They go to work, and before long all darkness is gone inside and outside people, except for one thing—the night. It is not long before those who remove all darkness can also remove the night by fitting everyone with special helmets that glow inside like the sun.

It is now agreed that darkness has been done away with—until it dawns on everybody that it still exists in crayons, paints, clothing, hair, skin, and myriad other things. So the removers of all things dark do it again: they manufacture a universal bleach that removes all traces of darkness wherever it appears.

The people are finally at peace: during the day the sun shines unblocked by any dark clouds; at night people wear their special sunshine helmets, and they can feel no trace of inner darkness (they take sunshine medicine for this, in tablet, capsule, liquid, and crystal forms); finally, universal bleach removes any remaining evidence that darkness existed.

Not long after this victory over darkness everybody stops eating, people stop talking to each other, and everybody disappears. The day this happens, dark clouds return to sometimes block the sun, shadows cast by buildings and bridges return, and one person who has survived gets those old feelings of irritability, anger, sadness, and dreariness. The special helmets don't work, so the survivor has to tolerate night and the pale moonlight. Dark colors reappear, for the universal bleach changed only the outer layer of things.

After the lonely survivor gets used to dark clouds, dark feelings, dark colors, dark shadows, and the darkness of night, things don't seem so bad. Before long all the people return. "Where have you been?" asks the survivor. "To see the dark side of the moon!" they all reply. They all applaud and hug each other, and as they do, the dark cloud moves just enough to let the sun shine through brighter than ever before, which creates the darkest, most beautiful shadows the people have ever seen, and when the night comes they play in the moonlight.

Now whenever dark feelings block their loving hearts, they wait for the shadows and for the moonlight, knowing soon it will all pass and the sunshine of their love will be brighter and more beautiful than anything they had known before. The darkness removers change their job description to read, "We only push the dark clouds a little to the left or right. We help you enjoy the companionship of the shadows. We help you wait for the dark feelings to pass. We hand out crayons, paints, and makeup in hundreds of dark and light colors. We open amusement parks only at night. We help bring you sleep that is restful. We help you understand."

*The End*

7. Have students combine an essay, poetry, or a short story with a drawing, painting, or collage to complete the activity. For an essay, students might choose one of the following titles: "The Dark Cloud in Me," "What to Do about the Dark Side of Life," "A Parable about Self-Esteem," "Don't Be Afraid of the Darkness," "It's What We Do with the Darkness that Makes Us Feel Good about Ourselves," or "The Secret Understanding: Our Guide to Self-Esteem."

## Bonding and Empathy

Michael Talbot (1991) tells the story of a young girl who, after being hypnotized, could taste everything the hypnotist tasted, including salt, sugar, mustard, pepper, and ginger (142). Talbot, explaining how the world and all information from it exists as a hologram, asserts that emotions themselves are also stored holographically. He says, "It appears that it is the emotional intensity of such events that makes them more prominent in the holographic record, and that allows normal individuals to unwittingly tap into them" (203). What do hypnosis and holograms have to do with Doorway 4's focus on bonding and empathy as ingredients in the development of "feeling tone" that codes abstract knowledge?

Bonding with another person and with animals and other living systems (such as Earth) creates a bridge over which emotional traffic travels back and forth. Bonding also enables us to extend those emotional bridges to others. These bridges carry feelings that enable us to sense who other people are. If we are denied bonds with others, we are also denied the bridges that enable us to sense what others are feeling.

There are few people for whom the bonding and bridge-building process proceeds smoothly. Sometimes the bridges fall down or partly collapse. They are rarely sturdy, and only with time do they show the endurance that many wise repairs have created. The path from bonding to empathy is lived each and every day, especially for teachers.

Jamieson McKenzie (1989), superintendent of the Montgomery Township Schools in Stillman, New Jersey, says that empathy is one of the skills our educational agenda must address: "Closely related to connecting and puzzling, empathy combines the skill of understanding the vantage point of others with the value of caring about them. Empathy allows bridges to be built. It helps people pursue 'win-win' strategies. It identifies the common ground. It resolves conflict. It brings people closer together" (10).

In the teacher exist all the positive and negative symbols of each student's history of bonding and the empathy (or lack of) it produces. The teacher stands in the place of parents, peers, and the environment, reaping the student's emotional history every time class meets. The teacher's own history becomes symbolized in the students, and they also reap the teacher's affective history. Both student and teacher dance with each other, attempting to create some form of bond so that they can feel for each other and in that feeling open up to the curriculum at hand. Like the young girl in the hypnotic trance who tasted what the hypnotist tasted, students who establish a bond with their teacher begin to taste firsthand what the teacher is teaching. They develop a feeling, an empathy, for the teacher as the living mediator between themselves and a world of ideas.

Each classroom both creates and unscrambles holographic information. The feelings that are produced in the classroom do not disappear. They become, as it were, invisibly present and continue to develop a sharper image in each student and teacher until the classroom has consciously as well as unconsciously settled into a pattern, a design, a hologram that is brought into focus each day by the continued relationships and patterns of the class. A "feeling field" is generated, which in turn brings into focus another part of the holographic record, and what we might call accelerated learning, spontaneous creativity, immediate insight, or sudden problem solving occurs. If the feeling field or affective hologram created by the class lasts for a long time it becomes difficult to change. This situation is fine when the stored feelings are positive but not so good when they are negative or violent. In either case the roads to higher-order thinking and memory are either freely traveled or blocked. Doorway 4 is a holographic dimension, a kind of emotional holodeck (for those who follow "Star Trek"), that brings into focus information that is stored in the worlds of Doorways 1 and 2.

## An Activity to Discover, Create, and Develop Classroom Bonding and Empathy

The following activity is a spin-off from an activity used in high school home economics, psychology, and sociology classes. You can use the activity in some early elementary grades, as well.

1. Divide the class into three- and four-member families that have two parents and one or two other relatives (for example, grandparent, aunt, uncle) who live in the same household. Have the group decide upon an object that they will use to represent a child in the family. The child can be of any age.
2. Each family develops an autobiography. Each member gets a new first name and they all share either the father's last name or the mother's. They may combine the two in the hyphenated form, as in "Smith-Robinson." The most important details are the biographical information they give the child (age, personality, likes/dislikes, health, schooling, problems, successes).
3. Set up various events. Each family chooses one or more events for which they develop a response. Following is a list of possible events:

    - The family arranges a meal.
    - The child is sick.
    - The family goes shopping.
    - The family dog dies.
    - The family decides to help someone.
    - Someone burns a hand on the stove.
    - The family argues over inviting a relative to Christmas dinner.

- The family decides what to watch on TV.
- The family goes on a car ride.
- The family has to move.
- The family plans a birthday party for one of its members.

Each group dramatizes its event or events in front of the whole class. The nature of the class will determine the time you set aside for dramatizations. You may want to videotape the dramatizations. When each group finishes its dramatization, the members of the rest of the class ask specific questions of each family member.

4. When all the families have completed step 3, draw out of the family members statements about their feelings toward each other. Before the whole class, direct the family members to come up with five emotions they feel about each other and have them share these feelings openly with each other. Following the sharing, the rest of the class will ask questions and answer them as the family looks on.
5. Unroll a 6-ft-x-3-ft piece of white paper for each family. Supply crayons, markers, glue, magazines, paints, and other supplies for making collages and writing graffiti. Each family carefully produces a collage about their family. The family actively constructs its own history going beyond, if possible, the events that have been shared to this point. The collage might include statements about the family, drawings and designs that represent what family is all about, letters between family members showing their many loving and conflicting feelings, and various statements and visuals culled from resources that reflect thoughts about family life.
6. Each family "adopts" another family and writes a letter to it, filling the letter with positive feelings and suggestions and encouragement for continuing their family life. The length of the letters will vary depending on the sophistication of the groups. Some groups might be encouraged to include in their letters quotes from various thinkers that reinforce the themes the letters express. Each family reads the letter it receives to the class.

7. All the families get together to plan an in-class picnic. The picnic will include food, music, games, and dancing.
8. This step calls upon you to develop a means by which each student will reflect upon "What It Feels Like to Be Close to Someone" or "What It's Like to Have Feelings for Someone in a Family." You may suggest the following mediums or any others you feel are appropriate to your group: poetry, essays, audiotape, videotape, art, art and writing, letter writing, a team conversation reflecting on the bonding process and its effect on young people.

Emanual Swedenborg defines love as "[humans'] willing, and derivatively [their] thinking, and thereby [their] acting" (Van Dusen 1972, 61). One could interpret Swedenborg's definition by alluding to an old saying: "Where your heart is, there also follows thought, and where your thought is also follows action." Simply put, one's heart determines the quality of one's thoughts and actions. This statement seems to unequivocally assert the importance of the limbic system in the development of thought and behavior. The quality of one's emotional life also has a causal connection with one's health. "Social connectedness is so basic and vital to human health that it affects blood pressure, the incidence of heart disease, and the intimate works of the immune system" (191) state Robert Ornstein and David Sobel (1987).

We know that loneliness and the lack of friends, especially in a society that is high powered and prone to substitute consumption for love, has a long-term effect on people, especially if the absence of friendship starts in childhood. Teachers are in a key position to pay attention to the ability to bond and the empathy, love, and friendship that their students seem to have. According to Richard Flaste (1991), researchers have begun to help first-and second-grade children who lack social skills and are troublemakers develop their skills at building friendships (14).

There are too many teachers who still refuse to see limbic, Doorway 4 needs as an essential part of their charge as professionals. Unfortunately, these teachers carry with them a denial mechanism that implies, "If they don't come to me well adjusted, it's none of my business. I'm paid to teach my subject. Let the counselors take care of the problem." This attitude cannot but add to a child's problems. Teachers interact with the whole child and it is refreshing to see that more and more academic caregivers understand that learning and emotional well-being go hand in hand. These teachers have come to redefine their professional identity as one that is intrinsically linked with student affect.

## A Student Friendship-Building Activity

While friendships cannot be forced, they can be encouraged, or at least children can be given experiences by which they might acquire skills that help them develop links and maybe even friendships with others. The following activity is applicable across the curriculum and, like most of the activities in this book, ends with some form of higher cognitive expression through writing, art, and discussion.

1. Hand out the first set of drawings of facial expressions on page 138. Be sure that you explain nothing other than that you would like the class to spend a few minutes studying them.
2. Form two-member teams by placing all students' names in a hat and selecting two names at a time. If you have an uneven number of students, you may have 1 three-member team.
3. Each team is to divide the ten faces into two groups of friends. The students do not have to divide the faces evenly, but neither group of friends will have less than three.
4. The teams give each face a first and last name. Under each name, the teammates write a list of words that represent what the person behind the face is like.
5. Each team explains why they grouped the friends as they did.
6. Each teammate decides which group he or she would belong to. The teammates cannot belong to the same group. They will explain why and how they made their choices.
7. Distribute the second set of faces on page 138 and ask the class to study these faces.
8. Ask each student to pick the five faces that represent the friends in the group she or he would choose to belong to.
9. Each student names and characterizes each face as in step 4, then explains why she or he chose that face.
10. Across the top of the blackboard, list the letters of the faces in ten columns and list the names of the students in your class

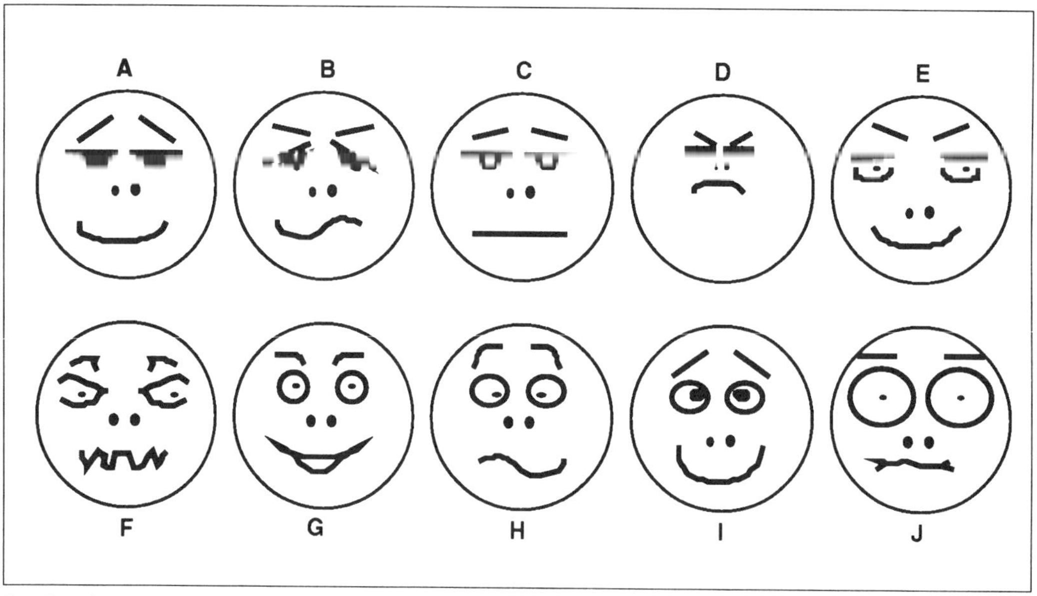


First Set of Drawings of Facial Expressions

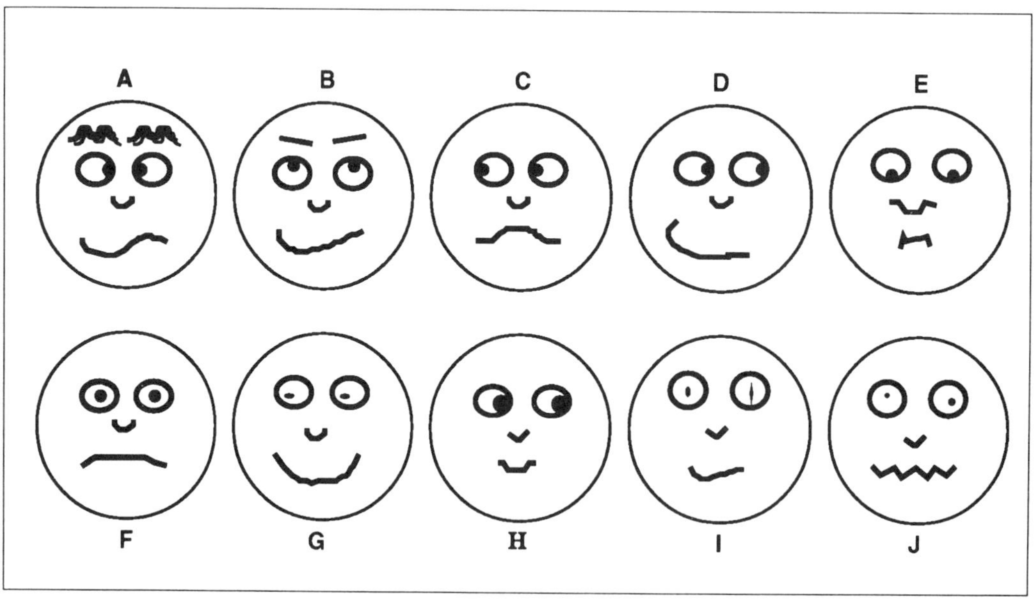


Second Set of Drawings of Facial Expressions

down the leftmost column. Ask each student to come to the board and, across from her or his name, place checkmarks under the letters that correspond to the five faces she or he chose as friends.

11. Use the results of step 10 as a basis for comparing reasons why more than one student chose certain faces. Also ask why no one or only one student picked a certain face. This exercise ensures that all the children will have at least one other student who has selected at least one of the same faces and shows that children share what they look for in a friend.
12. Group students according to the faces they selected, then give each group a problem to solve. Be sure that everyone contributes to the solution and that each child in the group can explain what every other member has contributed to the solution.

## Memory

Oddly enough, the limbic system plays a major role in memory storage and retrieval (see figure 5.1). While the words "storage" and "retrieval" have mechanical meanings, they are good enough analogies for the process we call memory. They suggest the act of choice, selection of storage location, motivation to access the information, and the possibility that memory may be lost due to changed conditions in storage containers.

The amygdala and hippocampus reside in the limbic brain. Facts, ideas, and emotions are stored according to their temporal necessity in either transitory storage or in long-term, semi-permanent storage. The hippocampus makes a decision depending primarily on the emotional coding given it by the amygdala. Strong emotional tags tend to route information toward the long-term storage areas in the brain. Other factors that tend to force the hippocampus into routing information into long-term storage are the following: (1) associational cues—the more visual, verbal, and emotional material that the fact, idea, or emotion is connected with, the greater the chance the memory will be retrievable over the long haul because more than one route to it has been created; (2) sensory stimulation—one physically acts out and senses that which is to

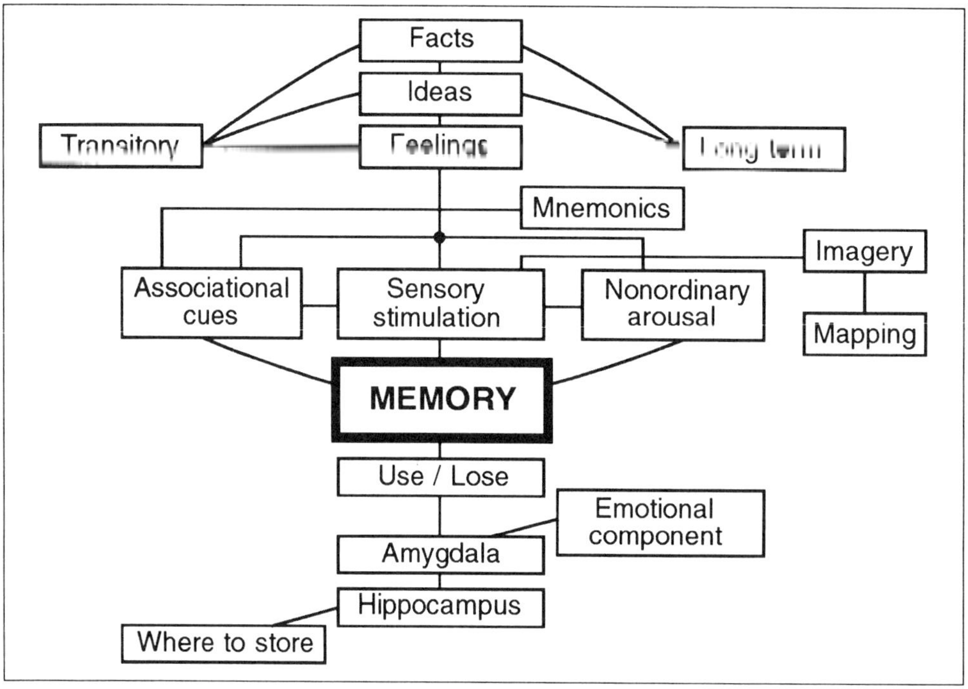


Figure 5.1. The limbic system's role in memory

be remembered, for example, builds a house in order to remember how to build a house; and (3) nonordinary arousal—memory centers tend to be activated initially by unusual experiences that in turn generate associated pathways that push information toward the long-lasting end of the spectrum of memory.

Following are specific techniques that involve associational cues, sensory stimulations, and nonordinary arousal.

- Mnemonic devices: We can immediately associate numbers, locations, acronyms, people, places, and things with what we want to recall. For example, words may contain mnemonic cues that we can use to memorize them. The word *compassionate* contains the word *compass*. A compass is a device that tells you what direction you are going in. You think of going in the direction of your friend's house. A friend is someone you love and care for, someone for whom you feel compassion.

- Imagery: Imagination and visualization allow the brain to create powerful, internal visual associations with items to be remembered. At least 10 percent of the brain is devoted to visual processes. Some researchers contend the percentage is much higher. Probably 30 to 40 percent of all students are visual learners. Except for a few students, visual associations create a very strong link with data. If, for example, a teacher wanted students to remember a chapter on the Civil War, he or she might do well to take students on a guided visualization of Lincoln's Gettysburg Address, including in the visualization all of the framework and details surrounding the event.
- Mapping: Nancy Margulies (1991) says, "When mapping, one is challenged to record ideas using not only words, but also symbols. In order to create a symbol one must use whole brain processing—words and images" (12). If you wanted to map this chapter, one possible map might look like the one in figure 5.2.

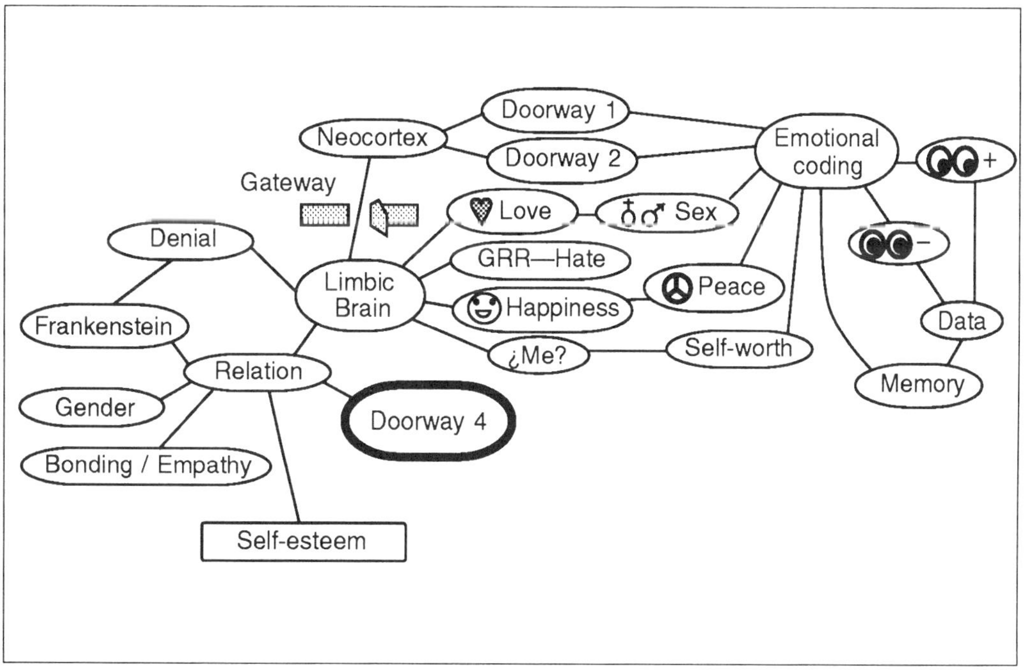


Figure 5.2. One possible mind map of this chapter

Memory itself is a fundamental aspect of Doorway 4 because our lives, our histories, are made possible not so much by what we remember but by the "feeling tone" that codes that memory. Had Mary Shelley's Frankenstein not been so alone, so bereft of love, bonding, self-esteem, and empathy, his memories would not have driven him to kill his maker nor caused him to drift away on a slab of ice into nowhere. Our students do not deserve the heritage of Frankenstein.

The power of feeling must inform or permeate the tightest of logic. As William Faulkner, describing the necessity of the heart's presence in writing, stated, "He, the writer, must teach himself that the basest of all things is to be afraid and, teaching himself that, forget it forever, leaving no room in his workshop for anything but the old verities and truths of the heart, the old universal truths lacking which any story is ephemeral and doomed—love and honor and pity and pride and compassion and sacrifice" (Augarde 1991, 78). The lesson of Doorway 4 is surely the wisdom of the heart.

# 6. ADMINISTRATION

*In a system of discipline, the child is more individualized than the adult . . . and when one wishes to individualize the healthy, normal and law abiding adult it is always by asking him how much of the child he has in him.*

—Michel Foucault, *Discipline and Punish*

Doorway 5 accesses the left limbic region, which deals with relational issues from a management or administrative perspective. When teachers laugh at the question "What does your child's room look like?" we know their Doorway 5 is active. Why is this question important and why does it provoke laughter?

When I speak of managing relationships, I am including relationships not only with persons, places, and things, but also with time, appearance, money, and other matters. Doorway 5 involves such issues as neatness, order, juggling the demands of other people, managing one's life, and administering the many details, data, and events of life. Focusing on the neatness of a child's room provides some information about the degree of activation of this limbic region in the day-to-day life of that child.

Most parents chuckle at the assertion that at some point children mysteriously become brain dead behind Doorway 5. Some parents even voice apprehension about entering the inner sanctum of their child's or teenager's room; they fear tripping over some ghastly object, animal, decaying food, or what-have-you. Of course there are some parents whose children keep a neat, ordered, and spotlessly arranged room. Such neatness says a lot about those children. What it says is neither negative nor positive but instructive, and as part of a complete package of related data it suggests what may work best with those children and in what areas they might need some help.

## The Notions of Order and Neatness

Maria Montessori (1966) writes, "A very important and mysterious period is the one which makes a child extremely sensitive to order. This sensitiveness appears in a child's first year and continues on through the second. It may seem to us slightly fantastic that children should have a sensitive period with respect to external order, since it is common opinion that children are disorderly by their very nature" (49). Montessori goes on to explain that this sensitivity allows children "to orientate [themselves] in the world" (55). The sensitivity is a child's way of maintaining the proper relationships between things and thus to connect with the natural order of things. The child is also able to locate himself or herself in this natural design.

Children also exhibit a second sensitivity to order that is connected to body awareness, specifically the patterns by which their bodies are handled. Montessori gives an example in which a child was bathed by two nurses. The child was pleased when one nurse bathed him but cried when the second nurse bathed him. The child preferred the way the first nurse held him while bathing him. The child's need for order extended into physical contact itself (57).

There does appear to be an inbuilt thirst for order in children and teenagers, yet Montessori more than implies that children are perceived as living in a disordered, chaotic environment. This mistaken perception probably comes from adults' own version of orderliness and their own internal sense of time and space. Adults often don't understand the kind of order children and teenagers live by and require. Teachers and other adults may not see the order within the apparent chaos before them, or they may not understand the rearrangements taking place beneath the surface disorder of a child's or teenager's room (or life).

As with so much we are learning about people, ideas, and structures of all types, order and chaos seem to be interdependent elements of reality. Order and disorder in some way feed into each other, always stretching toward some new order or arrangement. Doorway 5 houses properties within the learner that are paradoxical: they are interconnected structures of order and disorder, systems in balance and systems out of balance.

Understanding the rhythm of the fluctuations between these two halves of one reality is a difficult task. If a teacher is thrown out of balance by plans that are going awry, he or she is most likely not using the apparent disorder to develop the new order toward which the chaos is leading. Too often teachers attempt to impose an order on the disorder but only achieve another form of disorder, a disorder masked by order, a subtle form of repression.

To understand this most important paradox behind Doorway 5 we must take a look at what Ilya Prigogine (1984) has to say. After reviewing his comments, we will look at an important classroom activity that will bring Doorway 5 into clearer focus.

## Closed and Open Systems

To understand an open system we must comprehend what happens as a result of operations, actions, and behavior in that system. It is the nature of the open system that the elements within it change; the system is changed, sometimes slightly and sometimes radically, by the nature of the system itself. The elements should not be defined as permanent, since permanence is against the fact of the elements' natures.

Open systems cannot be treated as if they are closed systems without great damage being done to the elements or people who comprise that system. We must think about the classroom as an open system, not a closed system such as a clock, which is ordered by mechanical functions that repeat and do not change as a result of those functions. If classrooms were not open systems, education would be impossible. The exchange of information between teacher and student changes the student, and if the teacher is not operating repressively and mechanically, it also changes the teacher. One of the great problems with education and Doorway 5 is that an open system has been too often treated as a closed system. The results have been a continuing crisis in our schools and in our classrooms.

## Equilibrium

All systems have some form of balance; the elements work smoothly or happily together. This balance, or harmony, is called *equilibrium*. Sometimes the harmony is flawed by a minor dysfunction that upsets the equilibrium slightly; eventually the dysfunction may be corrected. There are times, however, when the harmony is seriously flawed and equilibrium is upset. This condition is called *far from equilibrium* (FFE).

In the FFE state, a system is most ripe for change because the slightest perturbation or the slightest behavior modification will send magnified ripples through the already unstable system, causing the system to enter a state of chaos, which may destroy the system or cause it to reorganize itself at a higher and more complex level. Prigogine called this self-reorganized state a "dissipative structure" because more effort is required to sustain it.

For example, as we learned in our chemistry classes, liquids suddenly reorganize their molecules when the liquid is heated to a certain level. Molecules shaped one way quite suddenly change their shape when the temperature of a liquid in an FFE state is raised even slightly.

Physicists themselves provide the perturbation that causes the system to change itself. The equilibrium within physics circles begins to break down when physicists change their intentions, revamp their definitions, and look for things unheard of in previous eras. A single physicist may suddenly add a new theory that causes chaos, and physics radically reorganizes itself with a resulting new concept of matter, time, and space. The physicist has changed and so has the physical universe.

In sociology, the same phenomenon occurs. The social order may remain fixed for years. People live within boundaries and layers of class, and dissension only slightly disturbs the order. Eventually, however, problems such as poverty, drugs, and prejudice reach a certain level and shake the substance of the structure beneath the semblance of order. Finally, in this FFE state, the social system begins to collapse. The system reorganizes itself into a new order or equilibrium. Such a reorganization is currently happening in South Africa.

The world of psychology brings our new understanding even closer to home. A person may live in a certain harmonious relationship with self and world for years, and then something happens. There is a death in the family, a divorce, a lost love, or a disease. The equilibrium is upset, and the individual experiences new feelings, new ideas, new hopes, and new despairs. The individual begins to fall apart, to suffer, and to let go of the old sense of self. In this state of disorder, the slightest idea or insight, or the briefest meeting with another person can trigger the emergence of a new sense of self. The person becomes self-reorganized and requires a new level of energy and connectivity to maintain the new harmony and equilibrium.

Finally, we see this process in pedagogy. A teacher may teach in the same way for several years, all the while hearing an inner voice that says, "It isn't working." At first the voice is muffled, not really disturbing the teacher's equilibrium or way of doing things. But over the years, the voice gets louder and the teacher's mode of operation becomes more threatened. When the equilibrium is disturbed in this way, the teacher may listen more closely to the inner voice and tamper with a classroom practice here and there while remaining uncommitted to change. Then comes that special conference, that workshop, that book, that discussion, that video, that something. This singular event is all it takes to shake the teacher, already in disequilibrium and ripe for growth, into a new level of identity, self-reorganization, and change. The teacher establishes new pedagogical order out of the chaos into which the old order was thrust. Most teachers understand this process very clearly and sigh a breath of professional relief that it happened to them and in them!

We have two seemingly contradictory assertions about order behind Doorway 5. Children require order; they also require chaos if they are to grow to another level or kind of order. The following classroom activity may help you understand the idea of order and also enable you to inject some chaos into your classroom in order to bring about something new.

## Classroom Activity on Order and Chaos

1. One day after school, change as many things in your classroom as you can. Following is a list of suggestions:

- arrangement of chairs
- your desk
- posters
- supplies
- the pencil sharpener
- the wastepaper basket

2. The next day ask your students to list as many of the changes as they can. Ask them to indicate which changes they like and which ones they wish had not been changed.
3. Divide the class into groups. The members of each group will compare and contrast the responses they came up with in step 2. Each group appoints a secretary who reports to the whole class.
4. Ask each group to reach a consensus on which change was most needed and which change should be changed back. The groups must be able to explain the reasons for their choices.
5. This step may be too advanced for some grade levels. Ask students to respond to the following individually: (1) state whether or not they felt good when they saw the rearrangement, (2) change one thing in the new format that would make a big difference, and (3) indicate whether they keep their rooms or spaces at home neat.

One of the benefits of this activity is that it gives you a sense of which students value neatness and which do not. This information will affect such things as how you give instructions, whether or not you type or print handouts, and even how you place a test on a student's desk. Sometimes your paying attention to students' needs for neatness and orderliness makes the difference between motivating a student or keeping that student interested and not doing so.

This brings us back to the seeming contradiction between the need for order and the necessity of chaos as a prelude to learning. After describing children at play, their randomness, skill, adjustments, roles, and rules, John Holt (1972) comments on the idea of structure and order in the classroom. He tells us that, although it is common to refer to certain kinds of classrooms as unstructured and others as structured, using these tag words "is a serious error. There are no such things as 'unstructured' situations. They are not possible. Every human situation, however casual and unforced has a structure" (9).

Holt's description of children at play reveals an innate structure or form that grows out of their common relations. Some teachers may also enforce a structure, while others do not. You can create many combinations from enforced structure and structure that rises naturally from the learning situation. How to balance creating order and discovering order in the seeming chaos of a given learning situation is one of the great challenges behind Doorway 5.

A teacher's response to the question of whether to impose classroom order ought to be influenced by the following question: Why is this order necessary? If the order is necessary to teach skills efficiently so that students can take their proper place in society, then it may seem sensible. If citizenship requires ongoing curiosity and continuing interest in social development and personal growth, however, then we may have to take another look at order; we should not use it to produce citizens who are merely cogs in the machine.

The administration of order and structure in our schools must meet seemingly conflicting demands of equilibrium and change. In his classic work on education, George B. Leonard (1968) points out this essential distinction: "It is not that the 'product' of our educational system is not 'capable.' He comes out with 'skills.' He may be a usable component in the social machine. But he is just about finished as a learner" (113).

The preservation of democracy may in fact require major changes in how we view the order that resides behind Doorway 5. Democracy is not preserved by an educational system that places all its bets on disproportionately imposed order, because placing such bets does not ask kids to choose, discuss, disagree, create, cooperate, and value curiosity and inquisitiveness. An order and a structure that nourishes these qualities, however, acts as the firmest, strongest, and wisest preparation for a healthy democracy.

Highly imposed order and structure tend to cultivate competition and the drive to acquire—two values, motives, and tendencies that place enormous restrictions on the skills and virtues necessary for the maintenance of democracy. These twin traits tend to inhibit a broad range of human development and to devalue some of the deepest needs human beings have regarding lifelong learning.

Alfie Kohn (1986) describes what most teachers have experienced. A child is the first to raise his hand to answer a question but forgets the question. The child's urge to compete overshadows the urge to understand what the question was intended to teach. To Kohn, this example illustrates that "competition generally does not promote excellence" and that "trying to do well and trying to beat others are two different things" (55).

A classroom structured around competition seriously blocks the idea that learning is an end in itself. The currently popular alliance growing between school and big business is perpetuating this competition. Much of the framework of this liaison defines the child as a potential wage earner, not as a learner for whom the process of learning is an end in itself. It is important that this emerging "partnership" not drown out the voice that says, "Behind Doorway 5 we minister to the structural needs of the child, not those of the business community."

Saying that a classroom is structured to help students develop skills to make them viable members of society is a euphemistic way of describing a competitive classroom where authentic learning may not exist. This simple fact, so pervasive in our classrooms, has kept thousands of incompetent teachers afloat in our schools for decades. Why? Because once educational experience is a means and not an end, teachers who have little heart, who have no grounding in the love of learning and the excitement of discovery, who don't value children as people, and who rarely have to think themselves, can latch on to an educational system and join the popular chorus of criticism that says the students have no skills. Such a criticism may be accompanied by years of fragmenting curriculum, of worksheets, of order in the classroom, of right answers, of objective tests, and of the same lesson plans year in and year out. What we determine as important behind Doorway 5 has profound meaning for the entire educational structure.

Competition is driven by extrinsic motivation (grades, material gain, and eventually work that pays well). The competitive pattern created in school programs students to enter an acquisitive and consumer-oriented society. In the long run, the inner senses are dulled, authentic voice trails off and becomes a faint and distant echo, and human beings learn to define their value by norms that are extrinsic (money, cars, houses, degrees, and profession).

It is no wonder that this process produces a society that, in turn, attempts to define what school is all about by producing formal, external, predetermined, and excessively controlling norms by which to measure what good schools do. Learning is very much an intrinsic process fundamental to the nature of the human person. This basic tendency is warped by schools and classrooms that remove this inner focus and use tools (created by people who have themselves lost the essence of what education is) to reshape the focus into artificial objectives.

The call to administer order in the classroom requires that a teacher, in time, come to terms with effective discipline and, typically, discipline that has as its sole end the control of student behavior. Discipline can never be so narrowly focused so that the administration of order becomes (a) a battle of wills and (b) destructive to inquisitive and creative learning. The greatest assurance that discipline will be effective, nonviolent, and nonpunitive is a classroom environment wherein what happens is interesting, challenging, and interactive. Herbert Kohl (1984) puts it this way: "Decent non-violent discipline will only be effective in a learning environment where interesting things are happening. There is an essential relationship between the quality of content and the use of non-punitive discipline strategies in any learning situation. Effective discipline is dependent upon building an attractive and comfortable world that children don't want to be excluded from, and not upon how you respond in any particular instance" (156–57).

The administration of order requires reevaluating what is going on in a classroom and understanding causal relationships between boredom and disruption. The onus must shift to the teacher before it is placed on the student. When the student has a chance to administer his or her own world order in response to situations that pique interest, that challenge, and that evoke participation, then the administrative role of the teacher operates in a framework of real justice. Only in this context can the appeal to student responsibility possess a persuasive quality that motivates self-reflecting and ownership of behavior that does not continue the whine of victimhood.

Children and teenagers thirst for order, but they also thirst for an array of accompanying emotions and attitudes. It is the wise teacher who has learned the path of Doorway 5, where order is understood as many faceted and as the balance between competing needs, only some of which are connected with the acquisition of traditional knowledge. The fastest way to create an orderly classroom is to listen to a child's need for order, especially when that child seems to be disordered.

The question of the administration of order nowhere raises its controversial head more than in how we determine who qualifies for special education and the prescriptive, pseudomedical way we determine the educational program appropriate for these students. It is no surprise that Lori and Bill Granger (1989) found that teachers think 60 percent of their students need special or remedial help and that a little more than 20 percent are handicapped and require special education (xi). It is surprising, however, that the Grangers found that one of every eight students is enrolled in a special education program (xii). Is this enormous and growing special education population a reflection on our basic problem with Doorway 5? Is it out of what we perceive to be chaos that we create these labels, these slots that will produce order and predictability in the school setting? In other words, do we use order-making to suppress the real needs of students?

Lori and Bill Granger (1989), with statistics and special reports to support their assertions, state quite frankly, "The truth is that most children dumped into Special Education—particularly full-time Special Education—are not helped any more than if they had been left in regular full-time classes and treated like ordinary kids" (105). Why are these students not helped any more in special education, and what does Doorway 5, administration of order, have to do with their not getting such help?

It may be too extreme to suggest that most special education focuses on the administration of order, but it is not uncommon to hear special educators cry for routine and predictability. Who hasn't heard it said that "kids in special education can't handle change"? Testing, individual educational plans, and the isolation of skill deficiencies that require remediation tend to create a bogus scientific-medical framework that makes special education classrooms look like a well-organized garage with cars that need tune-ups. We have created a system in which the wheels turn and the neat, orderly program looks good until one looks closely.

If the teacher is any good, all this pseudoscientific arrangement becomes irrelevant. Like any other teacher should, the special education teacher searches for what works and hardly justifies being labeled a special education teacher. This teacher does the work that should be done in all classrooms by all teachers. The line between regular and special education dissolves.

## An Activity to Dissolve Distinctions between Special Education and Regular Classroom Teachers

This activity requires special education and regular teachers to work together before including their students. The second part of the activity requires joining the classes in a cooperative effort to work together on a project.

1. Both groups of teachers gather and each teacher writes a response to the following questions:
    - What does a special education teacher do that a regular classroom teacher cannot do?
    - Describe the importance of the administration of order in your classroom and how you accomplish it.
2. Each teacher reads her or his responses in turn. Those listening take notes and develop specific questions to ask individuals after all have read.
3. Teachers ask the questions they developed in step 2 and discuss the responses.
4. The group brainstorms a list of what elements of order are common to the two types of teachers.
5. The group plans an activity appropriate for a class in which special education and regular classroom students are combined. One class of each will be combined, so if there are ten teachers participating, there will be five classes that will participate in the activity. The group also lists the ways that the teachers will administer order so that the activity will be a success. Each teacher will have a copy of the plan.

6. The group schedules and holds the combined class activity, making sure that in half the classes the special education teacher plays the teaching role and the regular teacher plays observer/evaluator, and vice versa in the other half.
7. The teachers will meet again and, when evaluating the activities, determine whether the line between special education and regular education has been partly dissolved. The group should deal with the question of whether or not the administration of order in special education classes is any different from the administration of order in regular education classes.

## Triaging Order

Doorway 5 suggests the administrative temptation to treat students the same way battlefield commanders and medics have had to treat the wounded. In recent wars the wounded were divided into three categories: those who could be treated and definitely saved, those who could be treated and possibly saved, and those who could not be saved and, therefore, should not be treated.

Sometimes this battlefield ethic takes over the world behind Doorway 5. There are those students who will succeed, those who may not, and those who are apparently a lost cause. Teachers do not necessarily conduct triage consciously, but the concept is pervasive in the teaching profession. To a great extent, the quest to order the educational system has caused us to produce various species of tracking and ability grouping. These tactics do not encourage higher academic achievement, but they produce a kind of order in which a teacher can expect to get on with things without expending extra energy to keep the peace. They produce in the student population a real sense that order and segregation go hand in hand.

The struggle to achieve order within a randomly created group is one of the most important experiences that we deny kids when we practice educational triage. There is an artificiality to an order that segregates according to norms other than those students naturally use to group themselves. The secret to the harmony required by the neural world of Doorway 5 is that students sense the healthiness of silence and focused, orderly activity when they are part of the process that produces the balance and the atmosphere in which they are swept away by the task at hand. All administration of order must at some point evoke a sense of value, a recognition that the order is useful and has been arrived at fairly.

## Doorway 5: The Doorway Out of School?

R. Buckminster Fuller (1979) produced many unified interpretations of an integrated, or what is called a cybernetic, world. It is a world aptly described as "spaceship Earth." It is a difficult task to take issue with a person who has discovered so much about how we learn, how systems feed back to themselves information by which to make appropriate changes, and how structurally and functionally interrelated all things are. It is hard to argue with Fuller's insistence that we need to develop a comprehensive understanding of life and leave details to the computer, with its ever-increasing capacity to store and ability to feed back specialized data.

In developing his comprehensive philosophy and understanding of the changing requirements of the role of education, Fuller (1979) suggests that schooling take place at home. He asserts that, with the available interactive technology, a student can really think and can absorb information at a faster rate in the privacy of the home than is possible in a school. Fuller makes a passing positive gesture to the social role of school but sees school primarily as a babysitting organization. He perceives both the home and technology as the ordering principles, or the administrative channels, for a structured education that will fulfill the needs of people on a planet that is changing quickly. Without arguing against either the home or technology as the proper avenue for the restructuring of educational experience and the reasonable response to a learner's need for order, I suggest that Fuller's overgeneralization does not truly reflect the power of a school, the enormous influence of teachers, and the needs of children and teenagers for an order that is worked out in an individual and communal way.

Fuller (1979) sets up his argument by stating, "I have taken photographs of my grandchildren looking at television. Without consideration of the value, the actual concentration of children on the message that is coming to them is fabulous. They really 'latch on.' Given the chance to get accurate, logical, and lucid information at the time when they want and need to get it, they will go after it and inhabit it in a most effective manner" (42–44). Based on this perception, Fuller says that teachers will begin to make video documentaries that will become part of an enormous pool of information available instantaneously to students through state-of-the-art technology. Fuller continues: "I would say then, that you are faced with a future in which education is going to be number one amongst the great world industries within which will flourish an educational machine technology that will provide tools such as the individually selected and articulated two-way TV and an intercontinentally networked, documentaries call-up system operative over any home two-way TV set" (51).

It is interesting to note that Fuller refers to Maria Montessori's method as a way of helping the child to focus to a greater degree. He believes Montessori's perspective on the child is mirrored in the incredible focus a child gives to TV. Fuller implies that the home, technical environment is equivalent to the influence Montessori's methods have on a child's need for order as an aid to focus on the activity at hand.

Fuller's praise of solitude and monasticizing of education in a people-free cybernetic bubble of technology requires consideration. We know that Doorway 5 requires a learning environment administered in an orderly way so that children can break through distractions and enter that wonderful place of unity between self and object. But does Fuller's forecast represent what is desirable and good for a child?

What happens to Doorway 5 under Fuller's view is that instead of housing the administrative potential for both communal and private organization, it becomes a hermetically sealed process of administering isolation from real people. It denies the communal dimension of education and relegates school to some sort of social exchange that has nothing to do with learning. Fuller suggests, quite ironically, that though children are connected to a planetary computer network, they can handle this connection only in isolation. Fuller's suggestions flies in the face of all we have presented in the seven doorways model, which proposes that learning requires both solitude and social interaction between real people, unmediated by technology.

The breakdown of the relationship dimension of learning creates problems related to the development of an orderly learning environment and is an approaching tragedy. How easy it is to isolate a child and provide that child with a technological interface. Instant order! But bypassing the sometimes messy and chaotic process of negotiating an agreement to support the need for order and harmony in learning is another way of insidiously controlling children and hiding them from themselves.

Relying solely on technology also communicates a message about consciousness. In the name of interrelatedness (the international computer network), this reliance teaches that consciousness is fragmented and isolated into as many parts as there are people who learn in isolation, befriended by interactive machines. "Consciousness," states Maxine Greene (1988), "involves the capacity to pose questions to the world, to reflect on what is presented in experience. It is not to be understood as an interiority. Embodied, thrusting into the lived and perceived, it opens out to the common. Human consciousness, moreover, is always situated; and the situated person, inevitably engaged with others, reaches out and grasps the phenomena surrounding him/her from a particular vantage point and against a particular background consciousness" (20–21).

The key phrase here is "inevitably engaged with others." If we want to organize and construct learning in little techno-boxes, then we might as well get ready for an Orwellian future wherein the administration of order becomes suppression. There is no consciousness in isolation no matter how much one is hooked up to the "outside world" via technology. It is in dialogue with each other that we truly discover the underlying structure of the world of others and of ourselves.

Greene (1988) explains that "the individual sees profiles, aspects of the building entered in the morning . . . aspects of the novel being read. As important, each time he/she is with others—in dialogue in teaching learning situations, in mutual pursuit of a project—additional new perspectives open; language opens possibilities of seeing, hearing, understanding. Multiple interpretations constitute multiple realities; the 'common' itself becomes multiplex and endlessly challenging, as each person reaches out from his/her own ground toward what might be, should be, is not yet" (21). What can we make of Greene's statements? Are schools, classrooms, and teachers fast becoming vestiges of a culture that is dying because technology is making highly personalized and individualized learning possible? Is the question of administering an orderly learning environment simply a matter of creating a cubicle of individual comfort supplied with enough tools and technology?

Perhaps the message here is that unless teachers reevaluate their profession, their profession will come more and more under the control of technicians. School itself is a corporate learning module where children are guided through programs, schedules, and personalities that far too often contribute to the chaos that invites commentaries such as Fuller's. Unless we come to terms with a new type of order, encourage debate and dialogue, and provide an atmosphere that teases the insatiable curiosity of youth, the technoplanners will eventually administer the order and harmony of a depersonalized learning process. Leslie Hart (1983) puts it this way: "Perhaps there is no idea about human learning harder to accept for people familiar with classroom schools than this: that the ideal of neat, orderly, closely planned, sequentially logical teaching will in practice, with young students, guarantee severe learning failure for most" (56).

Fuller's observation that the TV entranced his grandchildren seems to suggest that there is nothing else that can create this response. Yet how many teachers have witnessed that total engagement on the faces of children when someone reads a story to the children, when the children are solving a problem, when they are creating art, or when they are writing a story? Did Fuller see his grandchildren come and go from the TV? Such behavior is common. What might be considered rude behavior between humans is acceptable when we are in front of the tube.

That television is so venerated as an educational anesthetic by such a great mind as Fuller's is all the more reason for those who understand whole-brain learning and teaching to maintain an outspoken visibility. Imagine millions of students in isolation chambers being spoon-fed data as they interface with computers, whose mediated information is becoming more and more sophisticated—so much so that the real world may seem drab in comparison, lacking as it does the prefabricated perfection of the visual and auditory images supplied by computer networks!

## Recommendations

1. Ask students how they keep their rooms or their spaces at home. Their answers may be clues about what they are used to or what

they need in terms of the orderliness and neatness of the classroom environment.

2. Periodically ask your students what they like or don't like about the physical arrangement of the classroom. Their answers may help you plan for changes.
3. Study the patterns of as many aspects of your classes as you can. See if you can discover the orderliness or chaos designed into your class and the reasons for it.
4. Every once in a while jolt your class with an activity or an arrangement of the classroom that stirs your students out of their repetitive patterns.
5. Keep a thirty-day school journal that describes the changes you make, how your classes go, and your reflections on the changes. At the end of the thirty days study the journal to see if you can come up with one minor alteration and one major alteration in your teaching pattern that you think are desirable. Focus specifically on things you do to enhance the harmony and orderliness of the learning environment.
6. Once in a while hand out explanations for an activity and sit back and let things roll. Don't interfere (unless necessary) until the allotted time for the activity is up. Study the interactions, the accomplishments, and the failures of students. Follow the activity by discussing different questions about order and disorder and whether or not you should have intervened in the process.
7. Create an activity that requires group cooperation. The goal is for all groups to finish successfully. Not only must specific groups cooperate but they may help other groups finish the activity successfully. Discuss and take notes on what students say about the experience.
8. With a group of teachers, answer this question individually and discuss each of your responses: To what extent do you sacrifice the intrinsic nature of learning in order to administer and coordinate an "orderly" learning environment?
9. With a group of teachers, answer this question individually and discuss each of your responses: Do you think that your

classroom is attractive and comfortable enough that your students do not want to be excluded from the classroom itself?

10. Have a group of teachers from special education and a group from regular classrooms discuss the problems and philosophies of the administration of order in their classrooms. From their discussion, lead into a discussion of the Grangers' *The Magic Feather*.
11. Using the concept of triage, divide your most difficult class into three groups: (1) those who will pass; (2) those who may not pass; and (3) those who definitely will not pass. After making your list, consider what you can do to ensure that everyone passes and that the learning environment is orderly without being authoritarian.
12. Make a list of the positive and negative aspects of R. Buckminster Fuller's idea of an ideal educational experience. Be sure to consider the impact his vision would have on an orderly environment for learning. What kind of order is created and what is both good and not so good about it?

## Negotiation

Chief among the virtues behind Doorway 5 is the capacity to enter into a negotiating process the goal of which is the establishment of an orderly and harmonious learning environment. One of the necessities of this process is finding some kind of workable label that defines those around you, namely your students, but that does not categorize them or reduce them to that label.

If you are fairly certain of your vision of order in the classroom and you want to move closer to that vision, you can learn much about your students' response to your vision of an orderly, harmonious environment. According to Peter Block (1987), the key is to negotiate agreement and trust between you and your students. First you must identify where your students stand in these two areas, and for this purpose Block has advanced the grid in figure 6.1 (130–51):

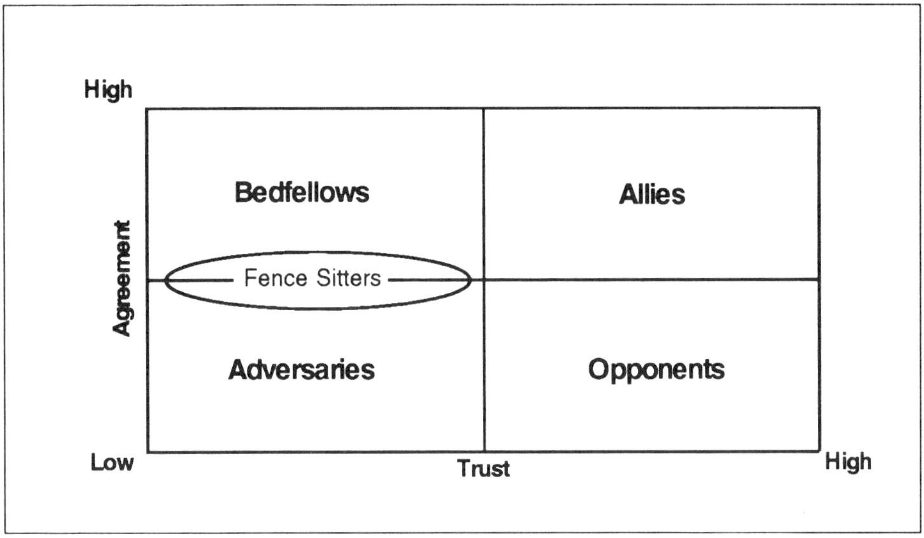


Figure 6.1. Block's grid for understanding students

The list moves from the most positive relationship with students (1) to the most negative (5).

1. Allies agree strongly with your vision of order and trust both you and your vision.
2. Opponents trust you but do not agree with your vision.
3. Bedfellows agree with your vision but don't trust you.
4. Fence sitters don't trust you and you can't discern whether or not they agree with you.
5. Adversaries don't trust you and don't agree with you.

It is in handling these different responses that your managerial domain is most challenged. Out of this potential for outer and inner discord you must negotiate an orderly and focused environment for learning.

This activity is not meant to make you the equivalent of a manager as portrayed in the business and corporate world. Administration of order is not a neat, tidy package whereby children and teenagers are "managed" or manipulated into position. Students are not clients you are preparing to sell something to. What they have to buy they already own. You and the student are collaborators in a process of discovery, and the road to this discovery, the process of collaboration, is like a marriage involving some agreement, some disagreement, some give, some take, some willfulness, and some letting go. Block's grid is simply a device to help you focus on individual students in an attempt to establish the ideal relationship with as many as possible. Block's grid is unique in that it requires the manager to be honest, to seek advice, and to be vulnerable with each type. The strategy requires spending a certain amount of time and effort with each type.

Allies are very important, and looking for new ones is vital. According to Block, "A well articulated vision statement and authentic behavior are the best way to find the support" (151). For you this statement translates to a clear communication of the kind of classroom you want, as well as just being yourself. Your next level of focus should be on opponents, because they speak well of you behind your back and provide honest, valuable information that might help you consider aspects of your vision and practices that you need to reevaluate. Bedfellows get the next level of attention; they need to sense you more personally, for while they agree with the vision, they do not have a firm bond with you. Fence sitters are beyond your control, and you can do little about them. They may or may not go along for the ride and on any given day may change like the wind. Adversaries, when not convinced of what you are doing, require you to communicate openly and honestly with them that your style is not working for them and that it might be best "to confess and say goodbye" (151). For teachers this confession translates to admitting the incompatibility honestly, without passing judgment or placing blame, and recommending that the student be moved to work with another teacher.

Sensing students' feelings and what is behind their attitudes and behavior can be either a science or an art. It is a science when it produces administrators who skate across the surface of categories and techniques of managing, organizing, and ordering children and teenagers. Such administrators' approach produces little satisfaction for the teacher and a kind of remote cooperation among kids. Sensing students' feelings becomes an art when administrators let go of this hyperrational, conscious effort to move things around. These administrators enter a flow of understanding and focus their efforts on a dialogue between teacher and student, and all see day-to-day life as sometimes black, sometimes white, and sometimes many shades of gray. This kind of administration strikes a balance between exerting control and letting go, between order and chaos, between knowing what comes next and not having a clue, and, finally, between concern for work to be done and concern for the young children who are supposed to be doing it.

The administration of order behind Doorway 5 is one of the most interesting tasks you must perform. The order must somehow emanate from your humanity and the meaningfulness of the curriculum in conjunction with the humanity of the students and their natural interests. Yet a secure, safe, ordered, harmonious, and balanced atmosphere for learning also involves a rational, willful, and sometimes conflicting set of circumstances in which you must use negotiating skills that may not yet have marinated long enough in your mind and heart. It takes time to internalize such rational approaches as Peter Block's grid. Don't rush into using such methods. Observe a lot, listen to yourself, listen to the students, then respond.

If you could tiptoe up to Doorway 5 and ask it for advice on the wisdom of administering personal and professional order, it might say what Rob Baker (1991) says:

> Balance itself is a more difficult basic concept to grasp than at first appears; it is something most people never think much about until they lose it. Almost everyone presumes that he [or she] has it—physically, mentally, emotionally. To question that would be threatening in a very deep, indefinable way. . . . But one has only to try walking down a rocky mountainside or to observe two children, slightly mismatched in weight, attempting to see-saw, or to remember trying to ride a bicycle for the first time—to realize just how delicate and discrete a thing balance really is, and how elusive it is, just like its close kin, harmony and peace, when we try to pin it down, define it, or hold onto it. . . . Perhaps the ideal balance is not a state of rigidity or stasis but is alive, changing, ever-shifting. There seems to be no easy formula for achieving or maintaining it. And once balance is obtained, it either degenerates into rigidity—a kind of rigor mortis—or becomes the impetus for new life, new process, new balancing, to being (23).

Behind Doorway 5 teachers and students together search for a balance, a harmony, an order. Getting to such order requires give and take. If the process becomes too tiring, you may fall into a heavy-handed approach. If you do so, rigidity will become the tenor of order in your classroom, your brain and your students' brains will eventually turn themselves off or, to survive, provide enough creative energy to play the game, mask the deep selves, and perform. But arriving at the state of balance and harmony means that together you and your students will begin the journey again with a renewed sense of trust in each other and a renewed sense of wonder; their creative energy will focus on finding their deep selves and finding wonder in the world to be discovered.

# 7. Motivation

> *Based on the false assumption that all students want to learn what is taught, the goal of most schools is to concentrate on both teaching and directing students without taking into sufficient account whether what is done is satisfying to students or teachers. Since none of the nonworking students are satisfied by this mechanical, pump-in-the-knowledge approach, this goal is rarely achieved. In fact, even many of the motivated ones do not do as well as they could. Test scores are low and will stay low until almost all the students, and many more teachers, find school satisfying.*
>
> —William Glasser, M.D., *Control Theory in the Classroom*

To want anything implies purpose. Purpose means that there is a goal or need that can be fulfilled. Sometimes you can meet your need or goal immediately. Sometimes you must go through a process to reach your desired end. The art of choosing both the means and the end involves a combination of abstract and emotional thought. To be deprived of one of these components in the act of wanting, choosing, and willing is to be denied the motivational basis for action.

One of the keys to teaching and learning is to understand the motivational framework behind decision making. This concept is available to us behind Doorway 6, which opens to the neural world of the prefrontal and frontal lobes of the brain. To understand this basic, inbuilt tool of the mind is to grasp the fundamental nature of motivation and the desire to learn. When we want to learn, there is practically no obstacle to learning. Teachers who can enter the domain of motivation can nurture it with their expertise, sensitivity, and knowledge.

Doorway 6 operates best in its forecasting function when the information from both hemispheres is complete. In figure 7.1, what verbal and nonverbal information is lacking that denies the farmer the ability to make an accurate forecast? Perhaps the information that is lacking is visual. He cannot see that there are not a lot of dark clouds. Perhaps the information that is lacking is logical. He may lack experience with dark clouds that don't result in rain. The final piece in this decision-making/ forecasting process brings us to the other important function behind Doorway 6.

Perhaps the farmer was not able to hear a kind of inner voice or speech that is part of a feedback loop in the language-processing function of the forebrain. Lack of this interior monologue, learned mainly through language interaction with parents, may dampen the higher thought processes connected with forecasting. Jane Healy (1987) puts it this way:

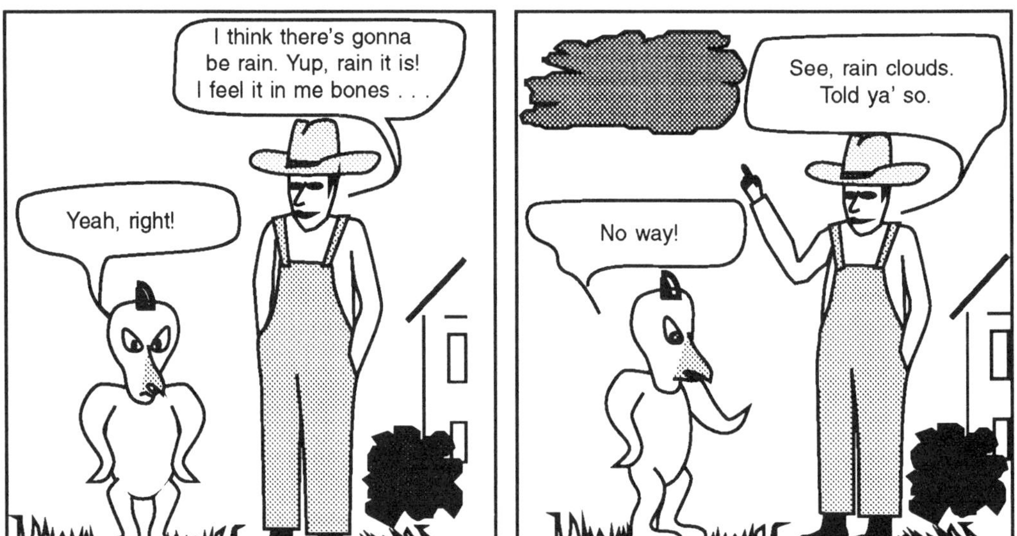
I think there's gonna be rain. Yup, rain it is! I feel it in me bones . . .
Yeah, right!
See, rain clouds. Told ya' so.
No way!

Figure 7.1. Problems created by incomplete information

"Can the use of language increase the brain's ability to think? Neuropsychologists now believe that 'inner speech'—the silent conversation that most of us carry on with ourselves—creates physical connections in several important parts of the brain. If you want your child to be a success in school, this ability may be the most important one of all" (193).

## The Role of the Frontal Lobes

David Loye (1983) uses Russian neurosurgeon Alexander Luria's description of his patients who have had lobotomies to illustrate the role of the frontal lobes in planning and motivation. Loye shows us that while these patients could think and act after surgery, they were able to use only those patterns they had established prior to surgery. The patients had lost their ability to plan for the future or to make new or creative connections between old and new information in order to solve problems. They were paralyzed when it came to acting on any postsurgery data and often performed bizarre actions, such as trying to light a candle by putting it in the mouth as one would a cigarette (58).

When the frontal lobes are confronted by a new problem, they quickly synthesize and analyze data from the external and internal world in order to get a working sense of what the problem is, what a person wants to do about it (goal), and how the person wants to solve it (hypothesis or guess). The person takes action, and if the action does not resolve the problem successfully, the brain fishes important data from feedback, refines or completely alters the hypothesis, and tries again.

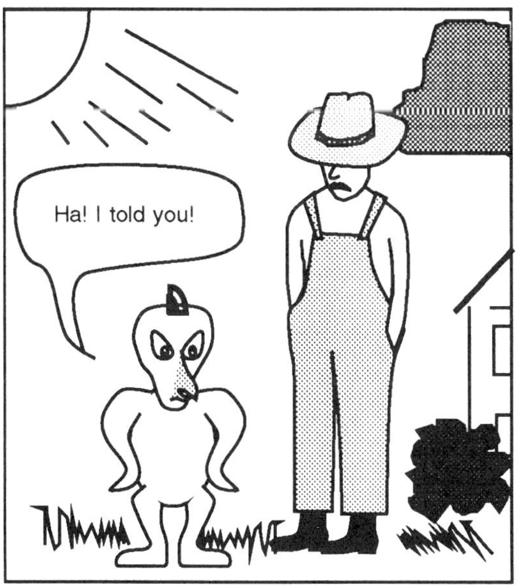


The frontal lobes, however, like all parts of the brain, don't work in isolation. Loye strongly points out the frontal brain's intrinsic neural relationship with the limbic and reticular (lower brain) systems. The limbic and reticular systems provide emotional, unconscious, and memory support for the plans being formulated at the higher brain centers. Lacking this internal feedback, the frontal lobes are unable to form a future sense. Current information cannot find a ground in the past or present as building blocks of the future, and the capacity to plan, guess, hypothesize, forecast, and act are shut down. There is no future and one is subject to the tyranny of past information and mechanical behavior based on it. One is bereft of the "why and how we are motivated to try to change the future to fit our desires and ideals" (60).

## Phineas Gage

We can get clues about the relationship of the frontal lobes to motivation by reviewing an accident that happened to a railroad worker, Phineas Gage, in 1848. An explosion sent a three-and-a-half-foot iron rod through Gage's head; the rod entered beneath his left eye and exited near his hairline. As the rod passed through his frontal lobes, it took with it pieces of brain and bone. Yet Gage lived, and seven days after the accident he was up and walking around. It became obvious, however, that Gage had changed.

Some of the characteristics people observed in Gage after the accident were childishness, obstinacy, irreverence, obliviousness to the feelings of others, and inability to stick to plans. He was unable to balance his behavior using both intellectual and emotional data. Having lost forever the relationship between his plans and the affective sense they would normally involve, Gage didn't know what he wanted, and when he did act to accomplish something he did so with a driven, tunnel-vision mania. He either did not care about something at all, or he cared with a singleness of purpose completely unplugged from human feeling. The latter is not really care; it is choiceless behavior rooted in neither like nor dislike. It is amotivational, a kind of schizoid separation of mind and emotion, devoid of purpose.

Gage seemed driven by childish self-indulgence and blind willfulness with no emotional grounding; he had little awareness of his own feelings or those of others. He didn't care what he was doing and was driven to act, as if possessed of radar that locked in to an action, blindly disregarding or simply cut off from feelings and judgment that could alter his actions.

He also would suddenly change plans, disregarding other plans as if they had never existed.

Richard Restak (1984) notes that lobotomies that sever the frontal lobes from limbic connections cause people to behave either as Gage behaved, blindly participating in purposeless activity, or sitting listlessly for hours without spontaneity or emotion (152). What can we conclude from Restak's observations about motivation?

It is important to see that Doorway 6 houses neural pathways whose connections to emotional, memory, and unconscious or automatic information ready a person to move into the future to achieve many types of goals. For the teacher this knowledge is another important link in understanding motivation. Because motivation is the readiness, willingness, and desire to do something, it is by nature a psychological state that is future oriented. Teachers are always presenting, eliciting, requiring, and even demanding work that is yet to be done.

There are three elements of motivation in learning. The first, affective investment, exists because interest, curiosity, and desire have been called forth. The second element, sense of control, occurs when the teacher and the students understand that the content, process, and product are co-owned, that students possess their own minds and the natural right to shape the curriculum with a shared ownership of direction and pacing. The third element is coplanning.

## Affective Investment

Motivation requires an affective investment if it is to be the driving force behind action. One must care about what one is doing. This care implies the continuation of motivation before, during, and after one has acted. The enormous satisfaction of a job well done is proportionally related to the affective investment. Gage apparently registered no satisfaction and, like many people, simply survived—in his case as a side-show freak in a traveling circus. He was cut off from the springs of deep feelings that make life worth living and his own life something to feel good about.

Doorway 6 holds one of the basic motivational secrets to learning. There is no greater motivation than that created by doing something one has a deep feeling for. "I really love school" is a statement equaled by no other for demonstrating a child's readiness to learn.

Daniel Berlyne (1971) defines the components necessary for this love of learning to occur: "To work at their best, the complex nervous systems of the higher animals seem to require a relatively high input of stimulation, excitement, and potential challenge" (412). To be stimulated, excited, and challenged requires coordination between feeling and action. In fact, this capacity to act because we find something appealing is one of the traits that separates us from computers. As Morton Hunt (1982) puts it, "Of all the components in human motivation, the one least likely ever to be simulated by a computer is our capacity to find things interesting. It is a mystifying phenomenon" (358). Neurological research therefore reinforces a basic and commonsensical fact: the classroom must be an interesting place to visit, and teachers must be practiced at evoking the natural curiosity of the child.

## An Imagery Exercise to Tap Motivation

Using the following guided visualization both students and teachers can begin to understand not only *what* motivates them but *why* the motivation exists in the first place.

1. As with all visualization exercises, each student should sit or lie down in a place where she or he is comfortable, a sort of chosen "sacred space." Have students close their eyes and relax by breathing deeply and concentrating on their pulses. Have them remain quiet for thirty seconds before beginning:

> *We live in the information age of TVs, VCRs, radios, CDs, video games, virtual reality, and computers. In this exercise you will be asked to converse with a computer to find out about it and to allow the computer to find out about you.*

2. Ask students to open their eyes. Show them the following designs:

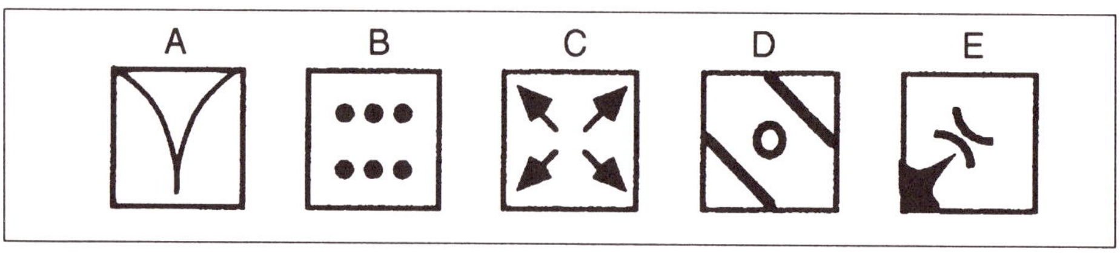

Have each student select the design that best represents the meaning or function of computers. Ask students to explain their selections. Then ask students to pick the design that represents a characteristic that a computer does not have but humans do. Ask for explanations and discuss students' choices.

3. Bring the students back to the relaxed place of step 1. Tell them that the trip to the computer is about to begin. Start the guided visualization using the story on pages 171–72, shaping it to fit your circumstances.

## *A Trip to the Computer*

*Imagine yourself walking into a tall building that has no people. Little computers control everything—the elevators, the robots that work in the building. The robots are dressed like humans, but they move about silently on a cushion of air. See the lighting and the colors, feel and smell the air, and allow your senses to notice anything else in this building. (Pause to allow students time to experience the building.)*

*Now look down a long hallway. At the end of the hallway you see a large, red, neon sign that says "McDonalds." You are hungry, and you walk down the corridor to the McDonalds. The door opens automatically. You walk to the counter and are greeted by a robot who cheerfully asks you what you want. You order burgers, fries, and a soft drink, but the robot asks again what you really want. You say something in return. What do you say? (Pause to allow children to think of something and to imagine themselves responding.)*

*The robot responds by telling you that you must take the matter up with Compubot, who is in charge of all computers and all robots in the building. The robot directs you to an elevator that is voice activated. You direct the elevator to take you to Compubot. You feel and hear a soft swish as the elevator rises to the top of the building. As you are going up, notice how you feel, what things look like, and what you expect Compubot to look like. (Pause.)*

*The elevator gently stops, the doors open, and you find yourself at the end of an enormous room. At the opposite end is a glistening brown table. A voice that fills the room tells you to step forward. You walk to the desk. Sitting in a chair behind the desk is something that appears to be a human being, except that tubes coming from the back of its head stretch for about twenty feet into a large mainframe computer labeled "Quadrant Six." Picture Compubot as completely as you can. See the colors and the material he or she is made of. (Pause.) Concentrate on how you feel: warm or cold, relaxed or tense, or any other way. (Pause.)*

*Compubot asks you what you want. You tell Compubot that you just want a burger, fries, and a soda. Suddenly, you understand. Compubot is not asking about food. You continue talking to Compubot, telling him about the things that most interest you. Compubot just listens with an occasional "Ah" or an "Oh, I see!" Take a moment to picture yourself talking to Compubot. Hear your voice as you tell Compubot what you want. (Pause.)*

*When the conversation ends, Compubot hands you a piece of paper that says, "You are lucky because you can be really interested in things and do things you really want to do, but I cannot. To be interested in things and to choose what you want to do makes being human such an adventure." You tell Compubot, "But you are interested in me!" Compubot replies, "Only because I am programmed to be so." Again you hear the voice that fills the room. It tells you that it is time to leave.*

*You turn and walk toward the elevator. As the doors close behind you, another voice says, "Get psyched, get stoked, get moving!"*

*The End*

4. Ease the students out of the journey and have them begin to free write. Ask students to include their lists of what they shared with Compubot.
5. Discuss the experience and develop a master list of what students told Compubot.
6. Have students form small groups and discuss how school is related to their interests and whether or not school is and can be an experience that motivates and interests them.
7. Role-play Compubot's conversation with a student and allow the rest of the class to ask questions.

## A Sense of Control

The next element in motivation is a sense of control. Neuroscientists believe that one of the most fascinating aspects of motivation is the relationship between the opportunity to exercise control over what is pleasing and the level of motivation a person has. In brain stimulation experiments with rats, researchers discovered that rats pressed stimulation levers more often if they were given a signal by which to anticipate a reward or if they were allowed to regulate the timing of the stimulations. Melvin Konner (1982) draws the following conclusion from these experiments: "In other words, the same stimulation could be very desirable, slightly desirable, or quite undesirable depending on the degree of subjective control experienced by the animal" (249). Konner's experiment echoes the human infant's joy in controlling external stimulation. Children who are interested in learning will tend to follow their interests when they have some control over the learning. Their need, desire, and choice to control are rooted in their motivational readiness.

The idea that a learner, already pleased by the teacher's presentation of content, might find that content undesirable unless allowed to exercise control over it would seem to be self-defeating, because the student would not learn something she or he is interested in. But consider what happens when a child does have control. The control allows the child to feel ownership of the content, process, and certainly the products of curricular life to a great degree. The child who is in control is a secure learner, able to grope this way and that to find out exactly what there is about the subject that is so interesting. The control allows the child to pursue various branches of information and experience within the larger content area at his or her own pace.

Learning is never just a matter of the child being a "blank slate" on which the teacher writes information. The child's mind is more like a chemical element to which the teacher adds other, complementary elements and helps develop. In fact the child may have been fascinated with the content before the teacher even exposed the child to it in the classroom. This phenomenon is known as "prior fascination," which suggests that the child is drawn toward reading, writing, building, playing, relating, and thinking because such activities are compatible with the child's inner world.

Teachers who share control with the students ensure that the learning process is not too predetermined. Too much predetermination and presentation of material contradict how the brain learns. The learning process by its very nature is codetermined through the wonderful conspiracy of student, teacher, and environment.

## Coplanning

Coplanning asks the teacher to involve students in some facet of planning what will be studied, how long it will be studied, and how what is studied will be evaluated. Students who help plan curricula exercise one of the most basic Doorway 6 aspects of motivation: plotting the future. If helps if you offer a variety of projects within each area for students to choose from. Offer ten to fifteen possibilities and require students to select five. Next discuss the amount of time students will need to complete each project and a due date for each. Be sure everyone agrees on this time frame. Finally, discuss the criteria you will use to evaluate the projects, fairly considering students' suggestions about what should be negotiable and what should not.

One of the more exciting aspects of such an approach to the curriculum is the possibility of serendipity, the discovery of unanticipated project possibilities that grow out of the students' other projects. Allowing your students to pursue such projects will teach them about firsthand experience and discovery, but you will need to renegotiate the time, due dates, and criteria for evaluating.

## Honoring the Intrinsic

From the earliest moments children attend school, most teachers use rewards to motivate students. Often, teachers choose rewards that are not related to the content or skill being learned. For many teachers, using reward systems is an ingrained habit and reflects the enormous impact behaviorism has had on education. Such teachers may see motivation as the relationship between that which is to be learned and rewards that await the accomplishment of that learning. Yet such a concept contradicts what we know about the neural reality behind Doorway 6 as well as observations of eminent educators, psychologists, and neuroscientists.

Jerome Bruner (1979) says quite directly, "Much of the problem in leading a child to effective cognitive activity is to free him [or her] from the immediate control of environmental rewards and punishments. Learning that starts in response to the rewards of parental or teacher approval or to the avoidance of failure can too readily develop a pattern in which the child is seeking cues as to how to conform to what is expected of him [or her]" (87–88).

Bruner continues by pointing to the development of all kinds of physical and psychological skills, the goal of which is to fulfill the innate need to interact with the world. Fulfilling the need has nothing to do with being motivated by extrinsic rewards. Establishing competence itself is the reward and the satisfaction. Children are curious by nature. They are by nature voyagers into the unknown. It is the process of discovery nurtured and guided by the sensitive teacher that allows children to reevaluate their knowledge and beliefs, to pass through cognitive dissonance created by previous knowledge, present discovery, and self-willed behavior into another plateau of cognitive harmony. It is important, according to Bruner, to allow a child to learn by discovery because "there will be a tendency for the child to work with the autonomy of self reward or, more properly, be rewarded by discovery itself" (88).

Michael Gazzaniga (1985) introduces the concept of "dissonance reduction": "Studies show that a behavior has to be strongly perceived as freely willed in order for the behavior to be powerful in participating in a belief change. Behaviors easily dismissed as carried out because of external forces do not engage the dissonance reduction process and as a result the belief system remains unthreatened" (141). "Dissonance reduction" refers to the relationship between belief and action. When action and belief are not consistent then "cognitive dissonance" occurs. For a belief to change as a result of an action, that action cannot be externally motivated, because external coercion will change only outward behavior; the inner belief, value, or reasoning process will not change.

To explain these brain-based concepts further, Gazzaniga refers to numerous classroom experiments in which children learn the same thing but through two different models: one that rewards the behavior and another that depends on the natural curiosity of the child. After students have completed the lessons, evaluators determine the frequency with which children voluntarily use their new skill. The results are quite clear: Those who are coerced by external stimuli rarely used the skill, while those who were not used it readily and often (141). Mihaly Csikszentmihalyi (1990) echoes Gazzaniga's findings: "I do not claim that most people most of the time act the way they do because they are trying to achieve goals; but only that when they do, they experience a sense of control which is absent when behavior is not motivated by consciously chosen goals" (242).

To understand the deep roots of human freedom, will, and autonomous goal seeking more fully, we can look at the relationship between choice and muscle movement. Sir John Eccles and Daniel N. Robinson (1984) describe studies of neural blood flow. They state that the first brain reaction caused by the intention to move is registered in the supplementary control area (SMA), whether or not movement follows. The SMA is not downline from any other neural area. Therefore, it appears that a mental event, or intention, acts on a neural location before actual movement, which occurs when the SMA links up with motor neurons. In people who cannot move, the SMA still registers their intention to do so. We have at the most basic level of bodily activity evidence of a highly autonomous mental intention interacting with a brain location that is not immediately connected to the movement intended. We want to move before we move. Movement is not simply reflexive, not simply a response to stimuli that acts on our senses, sending information to the sensorimotor cortex, causing it to feed back to the proper muscles the command to move. No, intention often appears first, and the source of this intention that activates the SMA seems to be non-neural, perhaps a nonmaterial awareness which we might call a soul.

Behaviorism denies children's freedom to choose to move, yet we see here that even on such a basic neural level intentionality registers before action. There do seem to be strong empirical, psychological, and neural reasons for asserting that Doorway 6 is the gateway to human freedom, and this fundamental aspect of children's whole selves must be respected and honored, beginning at the muscular level and continuing all the way to abstract and creative reasoning.

## A Brief Summary

There is no greater ally to the goals and intentions of a teacher than a student who truly wants to participate in the tasks at hand. Motivated students bring to life the content of a curriculum. To address the motivational issues of Doorway 6 successfully, we need to remember four things:

1. Try to make things interesting so that children are aroused by what you present. If you do so, you will invoke their "affective investment" and set their readiness to explore and work.
2. Children want to exercise power over those things that interest them. If they do not have or are not given such power, they may not follow their interests through. Planning to allow students to have a sense of control is the best way to ensure that their affective investment will carry them into the many stages of a task, lesson, or project.
3. Negotiate all aspects of a project with students, including what is to be done, how much time will be allowed for students to complete the projects, and the criteria for evaluation. Be sure to allow for those serendipitous discoveries that may prompt students to change their original projects. Teachers should handle all negotiations with a sense of fair play and good judgment. Remember that negotiation should not water down the challenge of the assignment.
4. Human beings have basic freedom of choice over their bodies, even over what seem to be automatic movements. Intentionality and purpose pervade the total psychophysical nature of children, teenagers, and adults. Teachers can best serve this interior design of freedom and autonomy by appealing less to extrinsic rewards and honoring more the intrinsic motives in children. Children value and use best those lessons in which the children find intrinsic value.

## Discipline

It is difficult to realize that all student misbehavior has a purpose, an intention, a goal. Students who have little self-discipline find something satisfying in their misbehavior. They may even be motivated to misbehave by the factors discussed earlier. They definitely have an affective investment in their behavior. It is hard to deny the level of emotional energy invested in misbehavior, albeit much is negative. Misbehaving students feel in complete control over their actions, even though the behavior itself may seem out of control. Students have taken control by choosing not to meet the demands placed on them. Students may also act as conspirators, coplanning their episodes of acting out or misbehaving. Finally, the source of the behavior is intrinsic in that the misbehavior and the punitive response it elicits are ends in themselves, requiring no other extrinsic reward or recognition.

In essence, discipline problems are problems of motivation, self-governance, freedom, and power. Kids who act out choose to act out because doing so fulfills basic Doorway 6 needs. According to William Glasser (1986), "We always choose to do what is most satisfying to us at the time. If what we choose is consistently satisfying, we will choose it with less and less deliberation, but even if it is quick as a flash, it is an action, not an automatic reaction. Only machines react automatically" (19). In other words, all students, well-behaved or not, operate by choice; however, the actions of students strong in motivation may seem never to be separated from choice or a sense of satisfaction.

To begin to change misbehavior, we must try to channel the affective investment into positive behavior by presenting our students with projects that are interesting and challenging. We must nourish students' sense of control by inviting them to coplan our curricula and choose their own projects as often as possible. And projects we choose should be interesting enough and pertinent enough that students feel rewarded and competent when they complete the projects.

We can nourish affective investment most effectively by relating to our students. Students need to sense a real person who is not hidden behind a role or a set of curricular instructions. Some of the great moments in teaching come when teachers let down their guards and tell stories about themselves or others and elicit the same from their students. These moments bond teachers and students, and students will invest more easily in the more formal elements of the curriculum once the stumbling block of a distant relationship is removed.

Teachers who choose to use Doorway 6 frameworks for developing curriculum and motivating students will find themselves assuming different roles. Teachers will maintain their roles as central figures in the classroom and students will still respect teachers and seek their knowledge and experience. But teachers will take on different characteristics in their central role. They will find themselves helping, discussing and negotiating with, advising, and encouraging students who have "taken the bull by the horns." These activities require as much creativity as predetermining and dictating curriculum, but they are more intimate and change the classroom into more of a learning community. Such teachers will be able to shift responsibility for learning to students because the students will have more emotional involvement, power, and desire to work.

## Teaching Motivationally vs. Managing Motives

Glasser (1986) has much to say that reflects the four elements of motivation. Glasser's most important point is that students find most satisfaction in learning when they have control over their own learning processes. Teachers, according to Glasser, must become managers as opposed to workers. As managers, teachers oversee the operation of small learning groups in order to "redistribute the power to get more productivity" (84).

Unfortunately, Glasser frames the redistribution of power in factory model terms; he refers to students' work as "goods and services" and students' overall output as "productivity." He says that students, "like all workers, will only work hard if they see that there is some benefit for them to do so. It is up to the manager to figure out how to structure the job so that they can see this benefit" (85). In effect, the job of the teacher is to break up a class into groups with tasks assigned by the teacher and tasks negotiated in the groups. The teacher's role, then, is to troubleshoot and to see that the groups get where they are going. Concerning discipline, Glasser states, "cooperative learning cuts off discipline problems before they begin in the classroom. Students are moved on task which, from a discipline standpoint, reduces the need for classroom management" (101).

While managing cooperative learning groups in itself is a worthwhile role for a teacher to play, it is naive to think it is the only role or the only important role. It is also naive to conclude that such arrangements always work or that they always represent shared power. There is something about the idea of managing cooperative learning groups that suggests the manipulative structuring of experience that is at the heart of behaviorism.

The act of learning is not just a matter of developing collaborative skills in a group managed by a teacher. After awhile such a format becomes stale and is upset by anyone who wants to move independently in another direction. The possibility for a kind of group tyranny exists, and an ironic loss of individual autonomy is always possible. Learning is not always best done in cooperative learning groups, but cooperative learning groups operate best when they are one experience among many in a classroom.

Eventually, the art and science of teaching rest in a sense of vocation, a calling to transmit knowledge, to nurture the insatiable curiosity of children and teenagers, and to bring one's experience and life to the experiences and lives of those whose education you are there to oversee. Sometimes the greatest motivation is the excitement and expertise you express when you present a poem, an idea, a piece of music, a story, a scientific experiment, a work of art, or any of a million other wonders of life and the universe. A deep reality causes teachers to be enthused by it all, excited by the opportunity to be there, manipulating nothing, simply satisfied with the work at hand. If teachers are intrinsically motivated, they pass their motivation to their students. Sometimes, the best motivation is simply to be there with what you love.

## Willed Not-Learning

The power behind Doorway 6 is enormous. It is what massive numbers of teachers face when students refuse to learn. These students fail but are not failures. They simply feel that their integrity, humanity, and dignity are not compatible with schooling.

In a wonderfully written pamphlet, Herbert Kohl (1991) describes case after case of students who decide not to learn. In each case the student is intelligent, willful, and most of all conscious of an inner worth that is being abused by society, represented by school. Kohl ends by telling us that poor and oppressed children will not stop rejecting school on a large scale until teachers become risk takers: "That means that teachers will have to not-learn the ways of loyalty to the system and speak out. We must give up looking at resistant students as failures and instead turn a critical eye towards this wealthy society and the schools that it supports" (74).

Sometimes the only way we can motivate students to begin learning what we hold out for them to learn is to face what is behind their resistance, their decision not to learn. Everything else will fail until teachers choose to set aside in certain circumstances their lesson plans, their power trips, and their management techniques. What has held education back is not so much the failure of technique or curriculum or system, but rather the failure of nerve, the loss of the enormous power behind Doorway 6: the will.

## An Exercise to Explore Motivation

The following exercise is powerful because all can participate, and participation takes only several seconds. The exercise involves three general steps: (1) Students act out a brief line, such as "I want to make something of my life!" (2) When all students have finished their interpretations of the line, they discuss a number of things, such as what the line means and whose interpretation they like most and why. (3) Students write a brief (twenty-five- to fifty-word) expansion of the dramatized line to share and discuss with the class. You will want to create some good lines for students to interpret in step one. The lines should allow students to explore some aspect of motivation. (4) Those who want to create an abstract design or other artistic response should be encouraged to do so. You will ask them to explain their visual response. Following is a list of lines that lend themselves to this goal:

- Nothing is gonna get in my way!
- I want it more than anything else in this world!
- I love this so let's have more of it!
- It's so wonderful I hope it never ends!
- Get the most out of school or you're a fool!

- I discovered I have so much to learn that it excites me!
- Jump in, get involved, and figure it out later!
- I've got to yell about it!
- Move over, Beethoven, the real music is about to begin!
- Go, Yo, Go, Yo, Yes, you gotta believe!

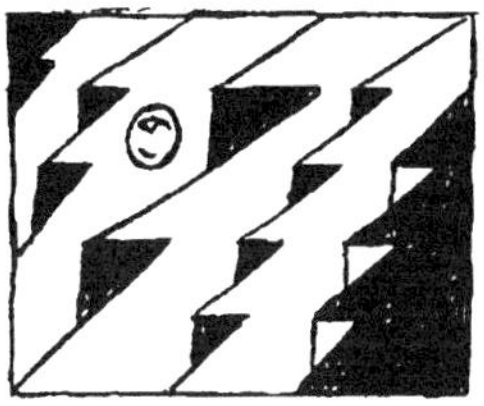

# 8. MOTION

*Life is rhythmic. It is through rhythm that we recognize the fact of aliveness.*

—Charles M. Johnston, *The Creative Imperative*

From many years gone by and out of memory banks dank and overrun by cobwebs comes a definition that was drilled into my mind. It is the definition of inertia: "A body at rest will remain at rest and a body in motion will remain in motion unless acted upon by an outside force." Isn't a teacher often that "outside force" that acts upon students, those bodies in motion that, if only they'd come to rest, would learn something?

Doorway 7 is, to say the least, one which opens to many problems, challenges, and possibilities. Doorway 7 is the sensory motor cortex and the area in the reticular system where the sensory, muscular, and overall motor systems of the brain are located. Motion is a behavior that is critical in the learning process, but many teachers simply have not come to terms with motion.

## The Quantum Key

In recent decades a revolution has been taking place in the field of physics that sheds light on Doorway 7 and the problem of motion in our classroom. For centuries scientists regarded the material world as fundamentally lifeless, obeying certain physical laws of motion automatically. Even after the discovery of the atom, physicists regarded atomic movement as just a smaller version of what one could see with the naked eye. Eventually individual physicists began to study the atom only to discover that what they were witnessing in their experiments was not what science had led them to believe should be happening.

This discovery caused a revolution in the way we look at the world. Elements in the microscopic world of the atom appeared either as particles (bits and pieces, nuts and bolts) or as waves (electromagnetic energy, invisible yet detectable force fields). Sometimes the tiniest structures acted as stable locatable objects, while other times they acted as if blown by the wind, suddenly losing their location and their objectness, and generating a certain amount of force. This discovery became known as the "quantum key."

As we explore the quantum key, think of the tiniest structures of matter as if they were students. Doing so will help you understand the duality that exists in the atomic and subatomic world. Students act in a stable, locatable way that allows us to treat them as we would objects on a shelf, placing them here and there, measuring them in such and such a way, and making plans for them. We can generally forecast certain outcomes based on plans we make for our students.

There is another side to students' nature, however. Students are neither here nor there; they are indefinable. Just when you think you understand them, categorize them, and plan for them, they seem to become invisible, unreliable, and irregular, and not only do your plans fail to shape their behavior but you can no longer forecast outcomes. Students, like atomic and subatomic particles, exhibit a clockwork predictability that can be planned for and around, as well as an evanescence, a mysterious quality of incorporeality, an energy that cannot and does not fit the neat categories of objectivity and measurability.

## The Three Quantum Paradoxes

Fred Alan Wolf (1981) describes three paradoxes created by what we call quantum physics. There is a universal web, or law, that motion follows, which includes the activity of the brain. Think of student behavior as you read the following anomalies; they will help you understand the world of motion that exists behind Doorway 7.

The first paradox Wolf describes is "things move without following a law of mechanical motion" (3). Motion, instead of describing a linear, point-to-point path, exhibits a nonlinear path with no predictable sequence. In other words, instead of creating a path from point A to point Z by going through B, C, D, and so on, motion may jump right from A to Z or from A to D or somewhere else.

Such a paradox resembles popular ideas about sequential and random learning styles. It suggests that students do not always learn by passing through steps but that they may take quantum leaps in their learning. It also suggests a connection between pure physical motion and learning.

The teacher and the students can cocreate an environment conducive to learning about each other by the way they handle rhythms of movement and location in the learning process. Teachers can interfere with their students' purely physical motion in two extreme ways: teachers can allow all motion or they can ban free movement in the classroom, limiting students to their seats. Of course there are many possibilities between these two extremes. But there is a relationship between how the teacher interferes with or disturbs students' motion/rest cycle and what the students will reveal to a teacher.

The second paradox is "[the instrument] one used to observe nature on an atomic scale 'created' and determined what one saw" (3). In some way the act of observing and the way one observes influences how the thing observed is going to behave. As a result objectivity is modified. What we see in anything is due partly to the tools we are using and partly to what we think we are going to find. In the subatomic world the tools we use disturb the world being observed and what we see is only a facet of the undisturbed world.

We can apply this paradox of objectivity to the classroom: students behave as they do partly as a result of the way we look at them, the tools we use to look at them, and what we hope or expect to find. In this sense we create their responses, and what we think we know about them "objectively" is really their response to the way we disturb their world. If we use conceptual tools that allow us to look for their original mind, their creative natures, we will most likely find them. If we use conceptual tools to look only for rote learning, objective answers, and respect driven by fear, these are what we will find. And yet because of the first paradox we may not get what we are looking for, especially if the way we treat students violates their deeply creative natures. In the final analysis, wise teachers understand the myth of objectivity and their roles in deciphering who the student is, what the student is doing, what the student knows, and what the student is capable of learning.

The third paradox is closely akin to the second paradox: "The order of the universe may be the order of our own minds" (Wolf 1981, 6). Our minds and the world outside our minds are really one reality. The world, then, becomes a mirror of our minds and our minds also act as mirrors of the world. Teachers often deny this capacity to change both mind and world. Unless teachers understand the quantum nature of reality, they will resist change and see this resistance create more resistance, which will require that more order be imposed.

It sounds simplistic but it does seem to be true that one of the major objectives teachers should have is to "go with the flow." I am not suggesting that teachers give in to chaos or abandon all control, but I am suggesting that the inherent interdependency between teacher and student will reveal to the teacher much more of what is necessary to unlock student potential. Teachers who fear losing control will become isolated from information that will bring them and their students to a new level of learning. On the purely physical level teachers must regard movement in the classroom as an essential part of the entire structure of learning, become more open to it, and learn what it means and how it contributes to all kinds of subject matter.

Ironically, the complement of motion, rest, also reveals what motion can offer the learning situation. Teachers need to stop resisting both motion and rest and understand that the two elements are integral to the unity of experience and, therefore, to learning. If such were not the case, most teachers would not be able to teach while moving or to sit at their desks and feed from this state of rest. Why have most teachers failed to realize that since they can teach while moving and resting, students can learn in the same way?

The secret for using motion and rest successfully in the classroom is in creating a balance between the two. Our neural networks run at peak efficiency when our brain-wave states oscillate between high and slower frequencies, between intense motion and equally deep rest.

## All Is Motion

You can't escape it. Everything is in motion. All human beings are sensorial moving forms that dance through space and time, oscillating between some form of trance and some form of conscious awareness. Children in kindergarten are sensing forms that dance through space and time engulfed in a trance, periodically conscious in a self-reflective way of what they are doing. In a real sense and without understanding it they are just being the motion you see. That is why it is so difficult to slow them down unless you engage their consciousness, enter the trance with them by using magic, storytelling, games, and so forth.

To get into their motion and to be able, as a teacher, to orchestrate it without crushing or discouraging it, you must communicate within the trance, the thought form that frames and drives students' bodies through space and time as if space and time never existed. If you teach in the early grades, you may want to imitate the movements you see among your charges in order to understand them better; you may get in touch with the thoughtfulness, the trance-minds from which students' movement originates. The learning-teaching principle is this: watch the motion, do the motion, embody it in a different motion (word motion, body language, slow motion, emotion, still motion), wait, watch the motion, and so forth.

The principle of imitating your students in order to understand them never changes whatever their age, ability, or the subject matter you teach. Effective seventh-grade teachers understand this principle intuitively. Unless you enter into the thought forms that frame your students' motion, you will never make contact. This making contact with students' multidimensional motion is the point of entry into their thought forms, which, in turn, helps you know how to approach them to help them learn.

Watch the motion and you will see incredible games of tag, unbelievable gangly arms and legs thrashing about, emotional roller coasters, notes sent-delivered-returned-redelivered in such a way that rivals the postal service. Watch all of this. Sense the abandonment and confusion of it. Imitate what movements you can. Feel how it feels. See if you can catch the thought there; yes, catch the thought there. Try to enter the thought in order to exit from it, to re-create it in word, image, story, emotion, and your own body language and facial expression. Then bring the thought back to motion by acting it out in puppet theaters, experiments, games, inventions, chances for apprenticeships in the community, and so forth.

The same relationship between motion, thought, and activity exists in higher grades. In fact the relationship continues in an idiosyncratic way throughout life. Not only do you observe the motion of groups to understand their structures of thought, but you also observe individuals in order to understand the nuances of thought within the larger group. Sometimes you cannot locate what you observe within the larger group at first, and you can only understand and respond to a particular person. You may find the latter case especially true if you teach gifted or emotionally confused individuals.

The idea that continual, never-ending motion is part of the definition of existence and applies to humans may seem strange, but this idea is a fundamental reality that changes everything we know about what Doorway 7 requires to make learning possible. From the subatomic level up through the human, everything is in motion and emits a certain frequency of sound and light energy. Everything.

Scientists have instruments to record the sounds of Earth, the beatings of our hearts, and the songs that we sing. Scientists have instruments that record the images of heat and reflections of light. We know that insects and animals see in the dark because of the type of energy they emit. The idea that all things emit energy leads us to what must seem the most esoteric observation of all within the context of whole-brain learning: all things, including humans, emit a song, that special sound or music that emanates from our moving parts, that orchestra of subatomic, atomic, molecular, skeletal, blood, and electrochemical rhythms and pulses that never cease to express themselves. All this motion produces sound and light, and it does so without our asking.

It behooves us as teachers to come to know this motion through its signatures of sound, light, and heat. We need to redirect our attention to the energy that announces each child's presence in our classroom. We need to watch the motion in all its expressions, including the subtle, in order to play curricular tunes that are valuable and useful to those with whom we are charged to spend a third of each day for a large portion of our lives and theirs.

## Play

If everything is in motion, then certainly a child's greatest expression is in his or her play. What do we observe in children's play, and can we transfer this playfulness successfully to the classroom and integrate it into the order, emotion, and rhythms of learning?

Catherine Garvey (1977) tells us, "Motion, the sensations of movement and the changing sensations that motion produces, are the first amusements adults offer to infants. Babies are jiggled up and down on the knee, tickled or repeatedly hoisted high in the air, and they show evident signs of pleasure in such experiences. And motion and changing sensations are also the first resources for play that infant[s themselves] can exploit alone during the time [they are] discovering [their] ability to control [their] movements" (25). Later Garvey tells us that these experiences are "enjoyed for their own sake and are divorced from other goals they might normally serve" (25).

In other words, in the earliest experiences of a child, motion is connected intrinsically to spontaneity, freedom, and joy, which serve no other goals than to encourage the movement itself. Movement is pure, original, and expressive; it is an end in itself, making it one of the strongest and most necessary needs within the human being. We must understand that motion itself demands our attention because it offers the possibilities of play, joy, and laughter as adjuncts and frameworks for all that goes on in a classroom. Associating movement and play with curriculum is a great challenge, one that we must meet.

What happens when play involves motion as children mature? Garvey states,

> In most cultures, play with motion for its own sake is joined with other aspects of play into more complex patterns. Rope jumping

> conjoined with rhymed verses; chasing and fleeing within a framework of social roles or themes such as Cops-and-Robbers; and group or team activities that have specified rules, limits, and sanctions, such as Hopscotch and Hide-and -Seek—all contain an action base of vigorous movement. In most human cultures play with motion does not disappear with approaching maturity, although it does come increasingly under the influence of social constraints and conventions that specify how, when, and by whom and in what garb the more boisterous and active types of play can be indulged. (38)

As children grow up their play becomes more socialized, more shaped by norms, more integrated with experience, and more complex. Part of the challenge facing teachers is to recognize this play and to associate it with classroom lessons and projects.

## Motion as Intelligence

It was Howard Gardner (1985) who seriously zeroed in on Doorway 7 as a true intelligence. Goleman, Kaufman, and Michael (1992) state, "It may at first seem odd to consider the body as the focus of a form of intelligence. After all, western tradition upholds a distinction between the mind and the body. But Gardner believes that the capacity to use your whole body, or parts of your body (like your hand), to solve problems or to fashion a product is as intellectually challenging an activity as figuring out cause-and-effect relations" (76). This statement sounds very much like what is suggested about the body behind Doorway 3, automation.

As a matter of fact, all people require some motion in order to learn. The type of motion and the amount of time that individuals need to learn optimally will vary from person to person. Some may require only a simple stretch or a deep sigh. Others may require a long walk to help them read, memorize, or discuss something effectively. Greek philosophers who created the idea of democracy were called "peripatetics" (those who walk around). It was during these strolls that they conducted much of their philosophizing and wove the ideas that structured much of the ideology of Western culture. Yet, in spite of all this, schools encourage students to sit passively in their seats while the teacher moves around.

## Ordinary and Unusual Ideas for Movement in the Classroom

You may use the following ideas for incorporating motion in the classroom in special settings, such as exams, or as part of the patterns of your classroom.

### *Final Exam Alternative 1*

Announce that at a certain time during the exam you will play the song "Dancing in the Streets" by Martha and the Vandellas. At that time students who wish to get up and dance may do so until the song is over. They can dance alone or with a partner. When the music is finished they must sit back down and write a given number of words on the topic, "How Life Is a Dance." They are free to use their written piece as extra credit or as a replacement for a question on the exam.

### *Final Exam Alternative 2*

About halfway through the exam, climb on top of your desk and ask anyone who wishes to climb up onto and jump off your desk to get in line. Explain nothing else until all who take your invitation have finished jumping off your desk. Tell them they may use the following assignment either as extra credit or to replace a question on the exam: Write a very short story about a child whose friends dared him to climb onto his teacher's desk during a final exam. The short, short story must contain the explanation of why the child chose to climb and jump and what doing so meant.

### *Final Exam Alternative 3 or Project 1*

There are a number of ways to organize the different elements of this activity. The most straightforward way follows:

1. Pick a poem, story, or descriptive piece and background music that reflects or enhances the literary piece you have chosen.
2. Read your selection to the class.
3. While the music is playing, present an interpretive dance or movement that echoes the meaning of the literature

4. After you have finished presenting the dance or movement, explain the connection between the movement and the literature.
5. Answer students' questions.

You can change the sequence of the elements easily. For example, you may begin by playing the music and presenting the dance or movement, discuss what the dance represents, read the literature, and finally, connect the literature to the previous discussion and the dance or movement.

*Final Exam Alternative 4 or Project 2*

Place pictures around the classroom to create a gallery, being sure to number or letter each picture. Students move from one picture to the other, viewing each without taking notes. When all students have looked at each picture, give them a handout with the number of each picture and space to write. They move again from picture to picture, writing down anything that comes to mind about each picture. As students are writing, you can mix discussion, art, and writing into the project.

You may choose to vary this activity. Choose pictures that are similar in some way: all animals, all children, all adults, all cultural artifacts. You will follow the same procedure, but the focus will change. For example, if all the pictures are of animals, the students might indicate how the animals remind the students of themselves. You can also create a museum experience. You can change the kinds of displays in your museum frequently depending on certain units, certain themes, and purposes of your curriculum. Central to this museum approach is movement and musing. Be sure to follow the activity with a visual, written, or dramatic activity, or with a discussion.

*Everyday Objects*

Organize your classroom so that students must move to get the objects they need to fulfill various academic and personal requirements. Such objects include passes, tissues, adhesive bandages, composition paper, and so on. The objects should not be items that students need permission to use, but the students should adhere to the general rules of respect, such as returning a bathroom pass in a reasonable amount of time.

## The Body Carrying the Mind through Space

Philip H. Phenix (1964) avers,

> The sense of movement is inherent in every human activity. To be alive is to be able to respond—to be moved and to move. All perceptions of the surrounding world are accompanied by motor reactions. Every experience, whether primarily of feeling, thought, or volition, engages the whole person, including the interconnected system of muscles, nerves, bones, tissues, organs, and internal secretions. No other instrument is as elaborate, sensitive, and intimately responsive as the human body. This is why the arts of movement are so important for the expression and perception of human meaning. (165)

The brain rides in a fluid housed in a skull that sits atop shoulders that ride upon a chest that rides upon legs, whose movement is balanced by two arms. The brain is a cowboy in a perpetual rodeo of motion or a spaceship hurtling through space, propelled by its appendages, which take it where no brain has gone before.

A child sleeps upon a pillow, but the brain hurtles through inner space in dreams, visions, and mysterious journeys. Upon awakening, the child moves all day through domestic, academic, and play rituals, carrying the mind through space via the body. This incredible and simple fact contains within it many secrets of the learning and meaning-making essence of the human being. Perhaps the fact is so direct, so simple, that it has eluded us. Well, not completely. We have physical and health education, drama club, and, depending on the level of school, dances, not to mention extracurricular athletics. Yet, these programs have segregated motion into the service of sports, good health, acting, and fun. Worthy as they are, these limited uses of motion tend to make using motion in purely academic areas seem out of place when, in fact, it is as integral to success there as on the ball field.

The essence of martial arts involves the body as carrier of the mind through space so much that mind becomes body and the duality is momentarily transcended. It is this fascinating unity that children and teens find so appealing and why martial arts have become popular after-school activities. While much of the attraction to the martial arts may be superficial, the martial arts give us further clues about the role of motion in mainstream academic education.

## A Martial Arts Learning Exercise

You may use this exercise at all levels of schooling. You need merely to commit to it, to reshape it intelligently according to the age and circumstances of your students, and to continue it intermittently over an extended time. Videotape the exercise.

1. Find a poem, an essay, a story, a math problem or process, a scientific or historical piece, or some other element of the curriculum that you want your students to learn about, read, discuss, and write about. Read it to them or allow them to study it.
2. You or martial arts experts instruct your students in basic body moves and the mental focus the moves require. (If you are uncomfortable doing this step yourself, you might want to invite the martial arts expert or teacher to do it. Teachers of tai kwando or t'ai chi ch'uan are good choices because these two arts require dancelike motion.)
3. Repeat steps 1 and 2 once or twice until you feel that your students' bodies are familiar with the moves.
4. Instruct students to combine steps 1 and 2. While they move through the movements, they will individually recite from memory what they have studied, describe what they have read, or answer questions about the material.
5. Divide the students into pairs. Each pair will go through the movements very slowly while discussing the assignment.
6. Show the videotape of the exercise to the class and discuss the tape.
7. Play an appropriate piece of classical music while students free write about the experience.
8. Have students share their writing with each other quietly, then ask volunteers to read their pieces aloud and to answer questions from the class.

This activity helps you and your students realize an ancient principle expressed in t'ai chi ch'uan literature: "In order to prolong the life of the body, to stabilize the life of the emotions and to intensify the life of the mind, conscious cooperation of the mind with activity is a deep necessity" (Delza 1961, 15). In the dance of tai chi the mind and the will focus on and move the body. This activity splits tai chi's focus and asks the body to share itself with curriculum content. The movement becomes an offshoot of tai chi, not strictly part of the tai chi discipline itself. You might want to use the martial arts movements as a prelude to study, discussion, writing, lab work, or other artistic expression in order to preserve the pure form of the discipline itself.

## Peripatetics

Derived from the Greek (*peri,* around, and *patein,* to walk), peripatetics originally refers to the practice Aristotle's students had of walking around the Lyceum while he was lecturing them. What could walking around have done for Aristotle's students to help them absorb and discuss his teaching and to develop depth and focus of thought? Some possibilities follow:

- Rhythmic and trancelike effects of walking free the mind from distractions and allow intense concentration on what is being said.
- The aerobic quality of breathing in fresh air maintains a steady supply of oxygen to the brain, which enhances listening, thinking, and speaking acuity.
- The two previous effects of walking would also open the mind to creative and unusual perceptions, associations, and insights about the topic at hand.

### Some Peripatetic Exercises

#### *Nature Walk*

Students follow a trail through a forest, a park, an arboretum, or a garden and carry writing tools and a notebook. At intervals, announce a topic such as birth, death, love, hate, freedom, democracy, school, and so on. The students stop and write about the topic for several minutes, then the group moves on. In a forty-five-minute nature walk the class might stop five to ten times.

You may make the process more interesting if you make topic signs and post them at various points along the trail. Inform the students that when they arrive at each sign they are to stop and free write. Students may want to continue their writing at some other time.

You can also use the stops to deal with various curricular content. A science teacher can prepare the walk so that at each stop the focus is on an aspect of the environment. A math teacher might have math puzzles set up at each stop along the way. A social studies teacher might place specific elements, artifacts, or writings that belong to a culture at each stop. The students would take notes about each element and move on until the nature walk has ended and they have amassed information and notes about the culture. Their notes would become the basis for later discussion and group work.

### *The Listen, Take Notes, and Talk Walk*

Students walk with you in small groups of five to ten. You speak on a topic for several minutes, then stop walking and talking. Students write notes from what they remember about your talk. After the students have written notes at the first stop, the tour continues. During the next walk, the students ask you questions about the first lecture. The group discusses the topic for five to ten minutes, then stops to write notes again. The lecture tour continues for two more stops. When the discussion ends, choose a new topic and begin again.

You can vary the walking lecture, note taking, and discussion in many different ways. You may take only three students and have one act as lecturer. Or you may have students walk and talk about a certain topic, tape their conversation, and play the tape for the class later.

### *The Blind Walk*

Divide students into groups of two to five. One person in the group will be the leader. The groups will go on walks, but only the leader will keep her or his eyes open. All members of the group hold hands and follow the leader across an open field or a beach while they audiotape a dialogue about curricular themes, topics, readings, events, and so on. Each group later plays its tape for the rest of the class to discuss.

### *The Sexes in Motion*

Girls develop small muscle control earlier than boys, and boys develop large muscle control earlier than girls. Gender differences in early muscle development contribute to sexual stereotyping and all the other gender-based biases that the women's and men's movements are trying to redress.

Females can help develop large-muscle control by participating in exercise, dance, and sports that use dramatic, large-muscle movements. Boys can help develop small-muscle control by participating in martial arts activities or other activities that require slow, muscle-area-by-muscle-area movement. You can incorporate any number of motion activities into your curriculum that will help boys and girls develop.

### *Sponge Balls*

Many sponge balls are available in toy stores. All teachers should have a variety of kinds and sizes on hand to use as part of discussions, tests, and games. Using them not only increases motivation but allows both boys and girls the chance to participate in body movement and to break down gender stereotypes males and females have about themselves as bodies and minds in motion.

One very effective time to use the balls is after the class has finished reading a story or completed a chapter in a science, math, or social science textbook. When all have finished reading, announce that you will throw the ball to different students, one at a time. Each student will catch the ball and do one of the following: answer a question; ask a question and toss the ball to someone else, who must catch it and answer the question; or begin a statement about the reading assignment and toss the ball to someone else, who must complete the statement. That person tosses the ball to a third student who adds information to what has been said and continues around the room. Of the many goals that are important here, one of the most important is that both boys and girls be equal players in the academic and physical aspects of the whole activity.

## Motion and Rest

Motion in an academic setting fulfills the need students have for random thought, the kind of spontaneous associations and perceptions that are basic to creativity. Motion shakes things up and when used well helps students bring to the surface of their minds all kinds of wonderful thoughts. The reprieve that teachers seek from the apparent chaos before them depends ironically on harnessing that chaos. Resisting the chaos and repressing children's natural urge to move is also to repress children's potential for discovery and their enormous capacity to come to terms with their findings.

Teachers use motion activities to invite a focus and an enchantment that leads to silence and total involvement in the task at hand. Balancing these complements is a science as well as an art. We best serve our students when we find and acknowledge these psychophysical structures in ourselves and recognize our own journeys into harmonic attunement. Then we can truly empathize with the Doorway 7 needs of students: the need of the body to move through space as a form of thought and the need to find nurturing of understanding and creative expression across the curriculum.

# 9. THE DOORWAYS AND OTHER MODELS

> *The idea that we have one rational mind seriously undersells our diverse abilities. It oversells our consistency, and it emphasizes the very small, rational islands in the mind at the expense of the vast archipelago of talents, opportunities, and abilities surrounding them.*
>
> —Robert Ornstein, *Multimind*

The 7 Doorways model is an umbrella structure under which many other models can be found. Before I explore the compatibility between the 7 Doorways and Myers-Briggs personality typing and Howard Gardner's theory of multiple intelligences, I must offer a caveat.

I once presented a workshop to teachers in a school system that had just finished an intense training in which the teachers studied the theory and practice of a well-known, whole-brain approach to learning. Although the model is a sound tool by which to structure curriculum and teaching, this group of teachers became polarized regarding how the program should be implemented. Half of the teachers wanted to test students to establish how to categorize each student according to the model. The other half wanted to allow the information to enrich their own sense of curriculum, teaching, and learning first and then to apply it artistically and intuitively to their classrooms and their students.

Unfortunately, because we are so influenced by pseudoscience, no sooner do we read about or attend a workshop on a new model of education than we want to create a questionnaire or a test that slots students into categories. This tendency to gather diagnostic evidence to establish a kind of prescriptive response is a cultural mirroring of the prevailing scientific model. This scientific model allows us to fool ourselves into thinking that we understand who a student is as a learner.

The purpose of the 7 Doorways model is to reveal the ways all people learn and the ways all people tend to behave based on an innate structure—the brain. The brain mediates the learning and behaving process, which is ultimately larger than neuroscientific evidence would lead us to conclude. The 7 Doorways model is a dynamic and generic model that neither reduces thinking, learning, and behavior to materialism nor attempts to suggest that the model is anything more than another pair of tinted lenses by which to get a view of the learning process. By making clear the explicit compatibility of the 7 Doorways model with the Myers-Briggs personality indicator and with Howard Gardner's theory of multiple intelligences, I am extending to these models the same perspective: They are simply lenses that enable us to view the mystery of human development and extract inferences about teaching and learning.

## Myers-Briggs and the 7 Doorways Model

The Myers-Briggs model begins with four basic pairs of personality indicators that reflect our innate tendencies in our interactions with the world:

1. *Extraversion and Introversion*. These characteristics describe the location or focus of one's mind. All of us tend to focus either outside or inside ourselves.
2. *Sensing and Intuiting*. These characteristics describe the source of one's thought. Our thoughts are based either on immediate outer sense perception or inner sense perception that transcends the here and now.
3. *Thinking and Feeling*. These characteristics describe how one processes data. On the one hand is the objective, sequential,

and cause/effect approach; on the other is the subjective and value-laden approach.

4. *Judging and Perceiving.* These characteristics describe how we approach situations. On the one hand is controlling, close-ended motivation. On the other hand is the flexible, open-ended rationale.

These pairs of opposites produce sixteen basic personality types. When we match these with the 7 Doorways model we get the following:

| M-B Temperament | Door 1 | Door 2 | Door 3 | Door 4 | Door 5 | Door 6 | Door 7 |
|---|---|---|---|---|---|---|---|
| ENTJ (Leaders) | ✓ | ✓ | | | ✓ | Closed | |
| ISFP (Observers) | ✓ | | | ✓ | ✓ | Open | ✓ |
| ESTJ (Administrators) | ✓ | | | | ✓ | Closed | ✓ |
| INFP (Servers) | | ✓ | ✓ | ✓ | | Open | |
| INTP (Problem solvers) | ✓ | | | | ✓ | Open | |
| ESFP (Mediators) | | | | ✓ | ✓ | Closed | ✓ |
| ISTP (Experimenters) | ✓ | | | | ✓ | Open | ✓ |
| ENFJ (Persuaders) | | ✓ | | ✓ | ✓ | Closed | |
| ESTP (Realists) | | | | ✓ | ✓ | Open | ✓ |
| INFJ (Inspirers) | | ✓ | ✓ | ✓ | | Closed | |
| ESFP (Live lifers) | | | | ✓ | | Open | ✓ |
| INTJ (Improvers) | ✓ | | | | ✓ | Closed | |
| ISTJ (Should doers) | ✓ | | | | ✓ | Closed | ✓ |
| ENFP (Energizers) | | ✓ | ✓ | ✓ | ✓ | Open | |
| ISFJ (Duty callers) | | | | ✓ | ✓ | Closed | ✓ |
| ENTP (Challengers) | ✓ | ✓ | | ✓ | ✓ | Open | |

I can illustrate how two basically opposite personality types relate to the 7 Doorways model. An ESTJ shows up in the 7 Doorways model as a learner heavily dependent on *motion* as the source of thought processes.

The thought processes focus on *causation* and the establishment or *administration* of an orderly existence, and the *motivation* for the processes is to establish a strict control over the ESTJ's experiences. An INFP shows up in the 7 Doorways model as a learner heavily dependent on *intuition* and *relation* as the source of thought processes. The thought processes are within the realm of holistic concept development, and the *motivation* for the processes is to help the INFP remain open to experience and an ever-changing or expanding conceptual understanding.

According to Gordon Lawrence (1984), among teachers "extraverts and introverts are about equally represented at all levels of teaching. The proportion of intuitive types increases as grade level rises. Feeling types are in the majority through high school, with thinking types outnumbering feeling types in college. At all levels judging types outnumber perceptive types. Administrators tend to have even more judging types" (21).

If Lawrence is correct, we can say the following about teachers and the 7 Doorways model: As many teachers are interested in the data/fact dimension of causation as are interested in the actual reasoning process and logical stringing together of that data within the world of causation. Between 51 percent and 61 percent of teachers from elementary through high school tend to focus on data that is derived from immediate sense experience, or **motion,** and that allows the **administration** of learning in a rather orderly way.

Teachers who rely on speculation or **intuition** tend to dominate at the college level, where they number between 60 percent and 65 percent. On the other hand, teachers in elementary and secondary grades show a heavy regard for **relation,** but teachers in college show a tendency toward **causation** or objectivity. Most educators, however, including administrators, exhibit a **motivation** to maintain a predictable, orderly, and planned environment. Between 63 percent and 70 percent of educators fall into this category.

In short, the Myers-Briggs statistics on teachers and administrators show a basic practicality in grades 1 through 12. Teachers focus on data and classification of data (causation). They prefer simple and immediate sensory experience (motion), which allows them to create hard and fast concepts (causation), all of which feeds their need for an orderly environment (administration). They show a sensitivity to **relation** and the values of their students, understanding the maturity level of their students and making room for mistakes. Teachers approach practical goals (motivation) that allow for measured success and control over all aspects of the school process.

The Myers-Briggs indicators reinforce what we think we know about schools—that they are places where Doorways 1 and 5 dominate. Understanding the Myers-Briggs personality types gives the teacher who uses the 7 Doorways umbrella model an advantage by offering another vocabulary and set of distinctions that can clarify the 7 Doorways approach. Conversely, the 7 Doorways approach clarifies the Myers-Briggs typology.

## Myers-Briggs and 7 Doorways Lesson Planning

The Myers-Briggs model complements the 7 Doorways approach by helping you ask yourself a broad range of questions when you are developing a lesson or a project:

- Do I understand that extraverts (E) prefer activities that include aspects of Doorways 1, 4, and 7? They like data. They like to talk with others about information. They like a certain degree of direct sensory input. Do my lessons keep these preferences in mind, and do my projects include these possibilities?
- Do I understand that introverts (I) prefer a higher level of conceptual understanding, that is, the use of analytical skills found behind Doorway 1? Do I realize that they enjoy seeing the relationships between things and are often metaphorical in their thinking? They enjoy some of the poetic possibilities latent in Doorway 2. They tend to search for the connections between things and enjoy this aspect of Doorways 4 and 5. They are often content to work alone or with another with whom they feel close. Do my plans and projects make room for them?
- Do I understand that sensing types (S) prefer action and the stimulation of their external senses in order to kick their thought processes into gear? Doorway 7, therefore, is of paramount importance to them. Keyed as they are into sensory information, a certain number of these types (especially if they are introverts)

might be aware of the subliminal sensory messages of the whole environment. For this reason the data available through Doorway 3 would be somewhat important to them.

Sensing types will not find the world of causation behind Doorway 1 important in its analytical, logical aspects. But they will find important its cataloging of data, which makes the tendency to classify of some importance. Do I take these cognitive needs into account when I plan my lessons and projects?

- Do I understand that intuitive types (N) prefer to establish the deeper meanings and connections in life? For this reason they combine Doorways 1 and 2 in an analytical search for the underlying, thematic, and symbolic meaning in things. Do I plan for these kinds of students in my lessons and in my projects?
- Do I understand there are thinkers (T) who prefer an objective, logical, well-reasoned explanation for things? They want depth along with precision. For this reason they indulge in the logical, sequential, analytical world of Doorway 1 as well as the orderly world of Doorway 5, where the administration of hierarchies and roles is important. Do I plan for these students in my lessons and projects?
- Do I understand that feeler types (F) require a great deal of room for personal and interpersonal values and free choice as the foundation of their thought system? What matters to them they hope matters to others, and, of course, others matter. Because others matter to them, their cognitive skills are heavily influenced by processes behind Doorway 4, relations. Do I plan for collaborative and group work as I plan my lessons and projects?
- Do I understand the judgment types (J) prefer the orderliness behind Doorway 5? They are goal oriented, thereby living in the motivational world of Doorway 6. Much of their cognition is driven by the desire for closure on what they do, whether processed in a sequential or an imaginative manner. Do I plan my lessons and projects to account for these types?
- Do I understand that perceiving types (P) are open ended and capable of adjusting to the flow of life, wanting to understand it as it happens, and not motivated by the lure of controlling it? Such

types tend to live in the relational world of Doorway 4. They also have a quality of sensory involvement that places them in the world of motion behind Doorway 7 and amid the flux that is ever present in that world. Do I plan my lessons and projects to account for these students?

Remember that the idea is to add a variety of lessons to allow all students to succeed. You will not be able to address every personality type's needs in each lesson.

### Matching Types with Types and the 7 Doorways Model

Theoretically, it may seem like a good idea to match students who are a particular type with a teacher who shares the same traits. Gordon Lawrence (1984) tells us that the following is a typical distribution of types in a classroom of thirty-five students: IS, 7; ES, 18; IN, 3; and EN, 7. ES types like to talk and IN types do not (40). Therefore, ES types will find classroom procedures difficult if the teacher requires a lot of quiet, individual work.

Since a higher percentage of students are ES types, teachers must come to terms with those students' needs. In others words, teachers must make Doorway 7 a dominant factor in planning lessons and projects. Teachers who will be most successful are those who are either ES types themselves or whose creativity moves them to develop lessons and projects requiring collaboration and a focus on the outer senses and inner senses of Doorway 2 as well as the kinesthetic world of Doorway 7.

All types, however, should also be challenged by their opposite types. Extraverts should practice silence, and introverts should practice collaborative group work. It is more important for a teacher to be able to plan for all types than to be matched with the typology of the majority of students in the class. The capacity to move in and out of all typologies and open all the doorways is a goal all teachers ought to be moving toward.

## Multiple Intelligences and the 7 Doorways Model

Howard Gardner (1985) introduces us to the theory of multiple intelligences (types of potentials and abilities). In essence Gardner takes the position that schools need to attend to the whole spectrum of legitimate intelligences, all of which are no less important and no less true than the kinds of intelligence that schools address and measure through standardized curriculum, tests, and intelligence quotients.

The seven forms of intelligence that Gardner identifies provide educators with another solid basis for creating an integrated, interdisciplinary, student-centered curriculum. The theory of multiple intelligences also works well with the 7 Doorways model. Each adds to the other a deepened sense of the model's meaning and significance.

## The Multiple Intelligences

Gardner divides the multiple intelligences into seven categories: logical-mathematical, linguistic, spatial, musical, interpersonal, intrapersonal, and bodily-kinesthetic. The first two, logical-mathematical and linguistic, are causal intelligences, wherein logical thinking and appropriate use of words are central. These are the intelligences most addressed by schools and according to which most teachers teach. These intelligences are classically left-brain abilities. In terms of content, we view them as maintaining an appetite for information, data, and facts. The classroom that focuses only on these processes can become a smorgasbord of lectures, rote memorizations, note taking, and testing for right answers.

The next two intelligences, spatial and musical, have traditionally survived only at the fringes of curriculum in spite of the fact that both are valid and valuable intelligences. Teachers rarely use music and art to organize their classrooms and design their lessons other than in a peripheral way. Although most early elementary schoolteachers cannot survive the daily lesson without incorporating music and art, these two elements gradually disappear as schools require students to exercise more abstract or formal reasoning.

The interpersonal and intrapersonal intelligences involve work between people and work within oneself. The interpersonal intelligence includes group dynamics such as leading, facilitating, cooperating, listening, questioning, summarizing, and tending to the overall emotional requirements and revelations within a group. The foundation of interpersonal intelligence is the interplay between the natural and nurturing forces of childhood and the bonding that must take place between children if this native intelligence is to flourish and become a force for creative growth. Without that nurturing and bonding, people can use this intelligence to manipulate groups and nations for dark purposes. The balancing of natural and nurturing energies can make or break the whole learning process, since the process is built on relationships that enable or impede readiness, on motivation, and on the willpower required for real learning.

The intrapersonal intelligence, on the other hand, moves students within themselves. This native potential is earmarked by an inner eye, ear, mind, and heart for one's own secret stirrings and the wish to maintain contact with them as well as to give them expression in the external world.

The last intelligence, bodily-kinesthetic, engages the body as the primary means of interpreting the world and giving form to experience. This intelligence parallels Doorway 7, one of the least-used potentials in the learning process in spite of its power. Most important learning events involve movement; for example, there are the sensorimotor events of infancy as well as the insights during adulthood that occur only during long walks, hikes, or strolls through parks.

## Building the Integrated Model

The relationship between Gardner's multiple intelligences and the 7 Doorways model is a natural one. The two models share four basic learning schemas: the analytic, the holistic, the psychological, and the somatic (see figure 9.1).

Both models also recognize that motivation is the master key to learning. Motivation is sparked when a teacher respects the seven intelligences and nurtures each in the classroom. When a teacher exhibits this respect, the purposeful and motivational door located in the frontal lobes of the brain swings wide open and the neural seat of willing, opting, decision making, and goal setting fires its electrochemical pulses, releasing the driving forces and energies behind all lifelong learning.

### *Schema A: Analytic*

Both the logical-mathematical and the linguistic intelligences rely on words. These intelligences revere abstractions only if those abstractions are tightly regulated by the laws of logic and empirical verification.

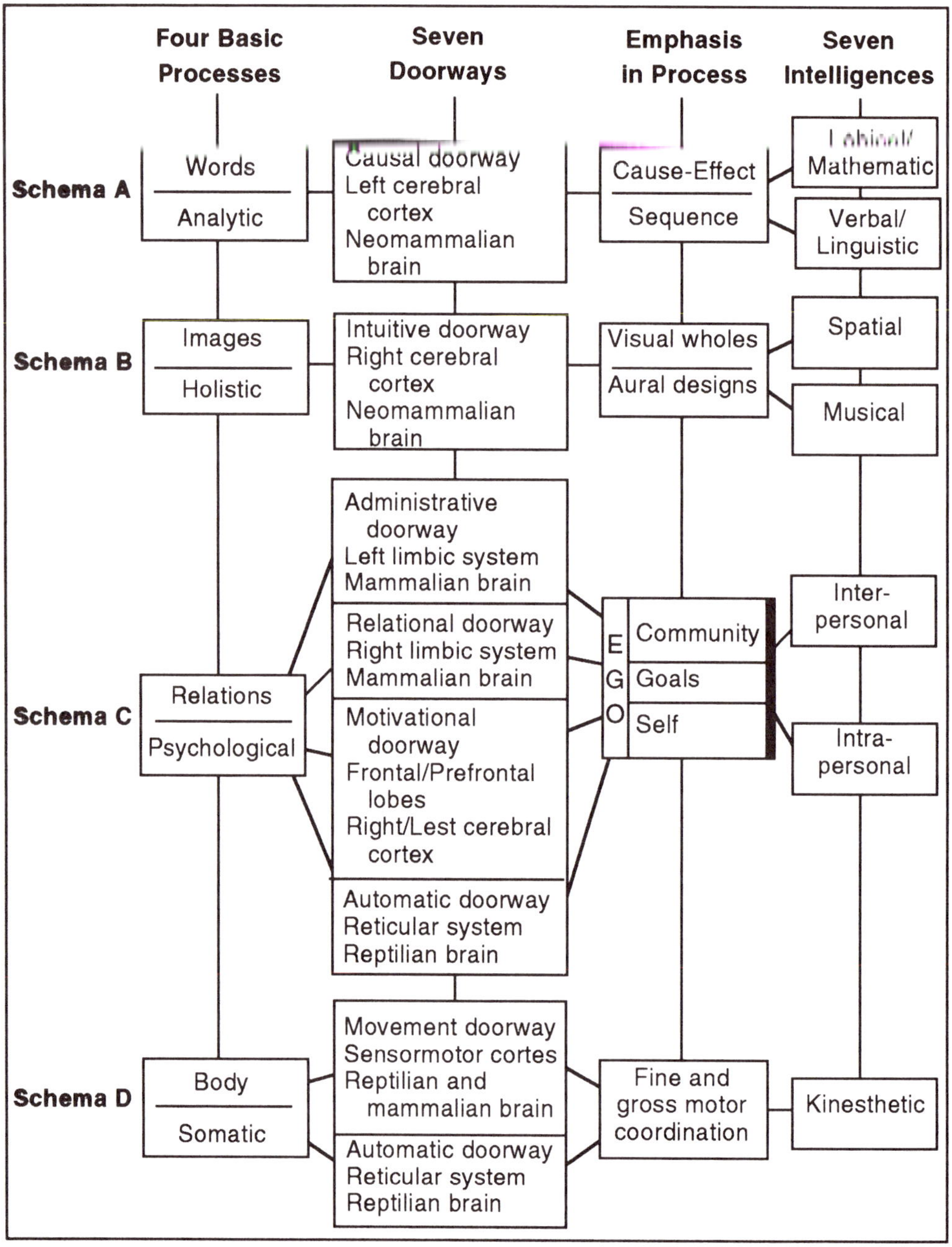


Figure 9.1. The four schemas: Diagram of the integrated schema

Organization and structure of thought and language are paramount. It is easy to see how these intelligences require great activity behind the causal doorway of the brain. Activities, projects, and tests that require the use of logic, reasoning, analytical manipulation of data (breaking data into its component parts), scientific proof, organized and grammatically correct writing, and the mastery of writing forms (poetry, essay, short story, and so on) all fall within this domain.

### *Schema B: Holistic*

The spatial and musical intelligences rely on imagery in the external and internal worlds. In the outer world, spatial ability involves the manipulation of color, shape, and texture. Musical ability involves the manipulation of sound to create music that is pleasing to the ear of the artist (and is only secondarily derived from the mathematical structure behind all sound). In the inner world, spatial ability involves the forms and appearances that rise from the imagination, as well as the development of internal visual states of mind. The inner world is also the place where the "inner ear" tunes in to "the music of the spheres." Activities, projects, and tests that challenge students to associate visual, auditory, and tactile imagery and feelings with words, both spoken and written, are central to the nurturance of these intelligences.

Nurturance of these intelligences must occur at all grade levels and at all levels of ability. It is through the spatial and musical intelligences that the authentic voice is salvaged in the learning process. These intelligences activate the intuitive doorway to the brain, through which holistic perceptions and creative flow from the unconscious are formed and channeled.

### *Schema C: Psychological*

The interpersonal and intrapersonal intelligences belong to the psychological world of the learner. The interpersonal intelligence involves the ability to work with others; to sense their feelings and thoughts; and to cooperate, lead, listen, facilitate, advise, counsel, problem solve, and set goals. This intelligence involves mutual nurturance and all aspects of relationships, including love and hate, sexuality and gender identity, and the process of bonding, which is the basis for the development of self-esteem. Interpersonal intelligence builds community by building the egos whose self-esteem is sufficient to withstand the rigors and rhythms of human relationships. It is a goal-oriented intelligence that seeks a vision of community and attempts to bring the community into being.

In contrast, intrapersonal intelligence is characterized by a heightened awareness of one's own feelings, thoughts, values, and judgments. The Socratic dictum "Know thyself" is sacred to this intelligence. It values and introspectively seeks out rich environments that are conducive to maintaining contact with the inner landscape of the self. Activities such as journal writing and the development of stories, essays, and inquiries that free the student to express the deep reservoir of the self are keys to opening to and using this intelligence. Respect for personal choice and for individual willpower keeps the energy of this intelligence positive.

These relational, psychological intelligences activate the relational doorway of the brain, or what is called the brain's limbic system. The limbic system is the most crucial of all doorways because it sets the emotional climate for learning. The relationships students have with themselves and with others will affectively code everything in the "official" school program. Without the positive element at the core of the development of these intelligences, learning becomes for the student a task that is empty of choice, value, and meaning. Lacking this positive affective energy, learning is based on a system of relationships built on authoritarian standards, legalisms that create order but disembowel true dialogue and wind up controlling feelings of negativity that fester beneath the surface of classroom interchanges.

Both intelligences also activate other doorways pivotal in learning. Interpersonal intelligence requires action behind the administrative doorway of the brain, which looks for ways to keep the external environment neat and the psychological environment of groups balanced. It tends to bring systems back to what might be termed homeostatic balance. Good managers know how to respond to individuals and groups in order to allow for a creative tension between their needs. This virtue is a hallmark of the administrative doorway in the limbic system and a trademark of people with the gift of interpersonal intelligence.

Interpersonal intelligence also opens the motivational doorway, which shares the neural circuitry of both the right and left neocortex in the frontal and prefrontal lobes and thereby coordinates and shares information from the right and left hemispheres. The motivational or purposeful doorway of the brain is the neural housing for the brain's function in the process of willing, choosing, planning, and goal setting. This doorway's activity is essential in the exercise of interpersonal intelligence and essential to group dynamics; when used properly and skillfully it assures both the individual and the group that sufficient analytical and intuitive information is present to make the best decision.

Finally, the motivational doorway is the seat of willpower, the energy that lifts an individual into an act of choice and ownership and moves one to lay claim to an idea or an act. In the case of education, it means laying claim to the work at hand because it is valuable and important to the student and to the group. We are likely to try to find solutions to problems that we care about. How many group activities fall apart for lack of willpower—the absence of resolve to get the job done diligently, intelligently, and with an ultimate creative harmony among its members?

Intrapersonal intelligence requires the arousal of the administrative and motivational doorways, as well, but it also requires the positive energy, feeling, tone, and sense of relaxation wherein introspection is natural. The introspective context is monitored by the automation doorway; the neural chemistry in the learner becomes altered and brain waves slow down to enter the meditative state wherein she or he can easily mine the raw ore of thoughts, feelings, and values. In conjunction with limbic processes, this state of mind fine-tunes the brain to a state of receptivity in which turning inward is natural. The physical environment is particularly important in stimulating this turning inward. Pillows, classical music, nonaggressive silence, and a general nurturing of inwardness go a long way toward tending to this intelligence.

### *Schema D: Somatic*

Kinesthetic intelligence involves motion. The movement and automatic doorways of the brain are important neural sites used in this intelligence. Pediatricians and other experts of child development have used fine and gross motor coordination for many years as criteria to measure normal growth and development in infants, toddlers, and young children, but coordination has never been addressed as an intelligence in its own right.

Some people are natural movers, using movement as a means of expression and a means of understanding, but all people require movement to trigger ideas and feelings. Kinesthetic intelligence is very alive in most students, particularly at specific developmental stages. (Ask most middle school and junior high teachers!) Yet in education we relegate this need to specialized classes, areas, and times of the day.

We know we must respect and nurture kinesthetic intelligence across the curriculum, especially in those children for whom it is a natural way of processing information from the world around them. These children are easy to spot; they move a lot. They move when they communicate and when they learn. In response to this kinetic impulse the most dangerous style of teaching is one that gives little freedom of motion. Besides repressing natural body energy flow, such a style retards learning itself.

## Gender, the Relational Doorway, and the Personal Intelligences

The importance of the personal intelligences in the total schemata of learning is nowhere more evident than in our increased understanding of the differences between boys and girls, particularly their patterns of human relationships and the impact of these relationships on their learning. The development of gender-specific interpersonal and intrapersonal intelligences revolves around two dominant and culturally reinforced modes of meeting the world: cooperation and competition. At a very young age boys are weaned from cooperative play to participate in competitive games, and their relational intimacy is cut short. Girls, however, continue in the cooperative, intimate mode until they are about twelve, when the same cultural forces that guided boys into competition earlier come to bear.

Having just come through a period when they can see what they see and speak what they want to speak without being penalized or losing their social bonding with other girls, females begin a period of intense crisis. Their need and biopsychological tendency to maintain close relationships and to define their self-worth through these companionships is threatened by social forces requiring that they begin to compete against each other, especially academically, for their place in the sun.

Because competition involves a new set of norms and pressures to conform, the adolescent girl finds herself at the horns of a dilemma: suppress authentic voice and belong or speak out and risk outsiderhood. It is an unfair choice, for she loses no matter what: on the one hand she gains intimacy at the price of her soul; on the other hand she gains her soul but loses her connections.

As previously mentioned, this entire process is remarkably documented by Carol Gilligan (1983). Because education has overemphasized the "right answer" approach to learning, it has also endorsed the competitive mode of interpersonal relationships and consequently contributed a great deal to the internal and social conflicts of students. If the gender-specific interpersonal intelligence of females leans toward cooperative, collaborative, and intimate learning, then classrooms must foster this intimacy and cease to participate in the social force that is destructive to the individual and society at large.

Such restructuring is important not only for girls but also for boys. Guy Corneau (1991) points out that an emotionally or physically absent father robs his sons of the male archetype necessary for boys to achieve a balanced relationship with the world: "It is the father's humanity that enables the son to conceive of a world in which things are not all black and white, and in which opposites can be juxtaposed and reconciled" (32). Corneau is saying that a father should play the role of helping sons achieve a noncompetitive relationship with the world, one in which it is possible to negotiate successfully through cooperation, colloboration, and intimacy. If in the best of social contexts boys become competitive at around age five, how much more they will become each year if they cannot bond with a loving, caring father figure. Because more and more boys are entering our schools from families in which a solid male role model is absent, it is paramount that we restructure classrooms to allow for a rebirth of the relational mode, especially through the presence of strong, caring, affectionate men.

On the other hand, true cooperation and collaboration must involve individuals who possess different talents and differing degrees of talent. Schools should not focus so much on group bonding that they suppress students' individual gifts and rights. The interpersonal intelligence, with its corresponding group dynamics coordinated by a teacher sensitive to female and male issues, should be balanced by the realm of intrapersonal intelligence, where the focus is within the individual and where personal thoughts, feelings, and values are nourished without fostering competition. This self-awareness requires expression, and work in the interpersonal realm makes this expression possible.

The theory of multiple intelligences in conjunction with the whole-brain model of the 7 Doorways offers a learning framework in which everyone can develop talents without fearing the loss of connection to the group. The development of talents and encouragement of healthy bonding are the most important reasons for using this approach to restructure classrooms.

### *An Activity from the Integrated Model*

The following project was given to students in tenth-grade English classes. Because the school, unfortunately, groups students according to ability, the project offered different activities and had different criteria for evaluation depending on the group's perceived ability.

What the students created in response to the project was truly amazing in depth and in interdisciplinary scope. Their presentations included live and recorded music, dramatic acting, poetry readings, dance improvisations, game making, and other equally fascinating offerings. All the activities were accompanied by a substantial written piece to ground them in the language arts and to make them legitimate in an English classroom.

Students grouped in the middle (level 2) love to work in groups but are less task oriented than the top, level 1 students. Group 2 presentations were good, especially since the activity required the students to create projects, one of which had to be presented to the class. To meet this criterion, the students had to break through the comfort zone of isolated group work to face the whole class.

Many of the lower-level kids (levels 3 and 4) did not opt for the more risk-taking possibilities of the activity and chose to stay within traditional verbal and linguistic patterns. There were some who did use the opportunity to expand their horizons and work with a teammate or produce art. The tracking system causes these students to expect less of themselves and the system, and they have been socialized to accept this lower expectation. As a result they don't want to appear motivated to respond academically.

I expected all students to perform well, and the project did elicit many excellent results. Certain teachers may have a tendency to focus on just a few of the intelligences when they assign the project and allow students to choose activities at random, but these teachers can counter their tendencies by structuring the project to continue for a long time and requiring that each student work on at least one activity from each of the seven intelligences.

To begin the project, each student was given a two-page handout that outlined and explained the integrated model and the requirements students were to meet. One page of the handout had a circular chart that reviewed the theories and offered students a choice among activities connected to each intelligence. The design in figure 9.2. was given to the higher-level group after they had read and discussed the classic novel by James Hilton, *Lost Horizon.* Each student had to choose one activity from each of five intelligences and had to participate in the preparation of at least one large-group presentation.

Needless to say this integrated model has enormous potential for structuring classroom life. You can set up a classroom with seven centers that reflect each aspect of the model. Students could concentrate on each center and move through them in a predetermined sequence or in an individually selected sequence. There are many possibilities.

## Conclusion

Two models of human perception and cognition have a basis in the whole-brain model of the 7 Doorways model. The fact is that all legitimate models of learning are grounded in the 7 Doorways model. Because the areas of teaching and learning are so grounded, we must consider the 7 Doorways model when we begin to reform and restructure our schools.

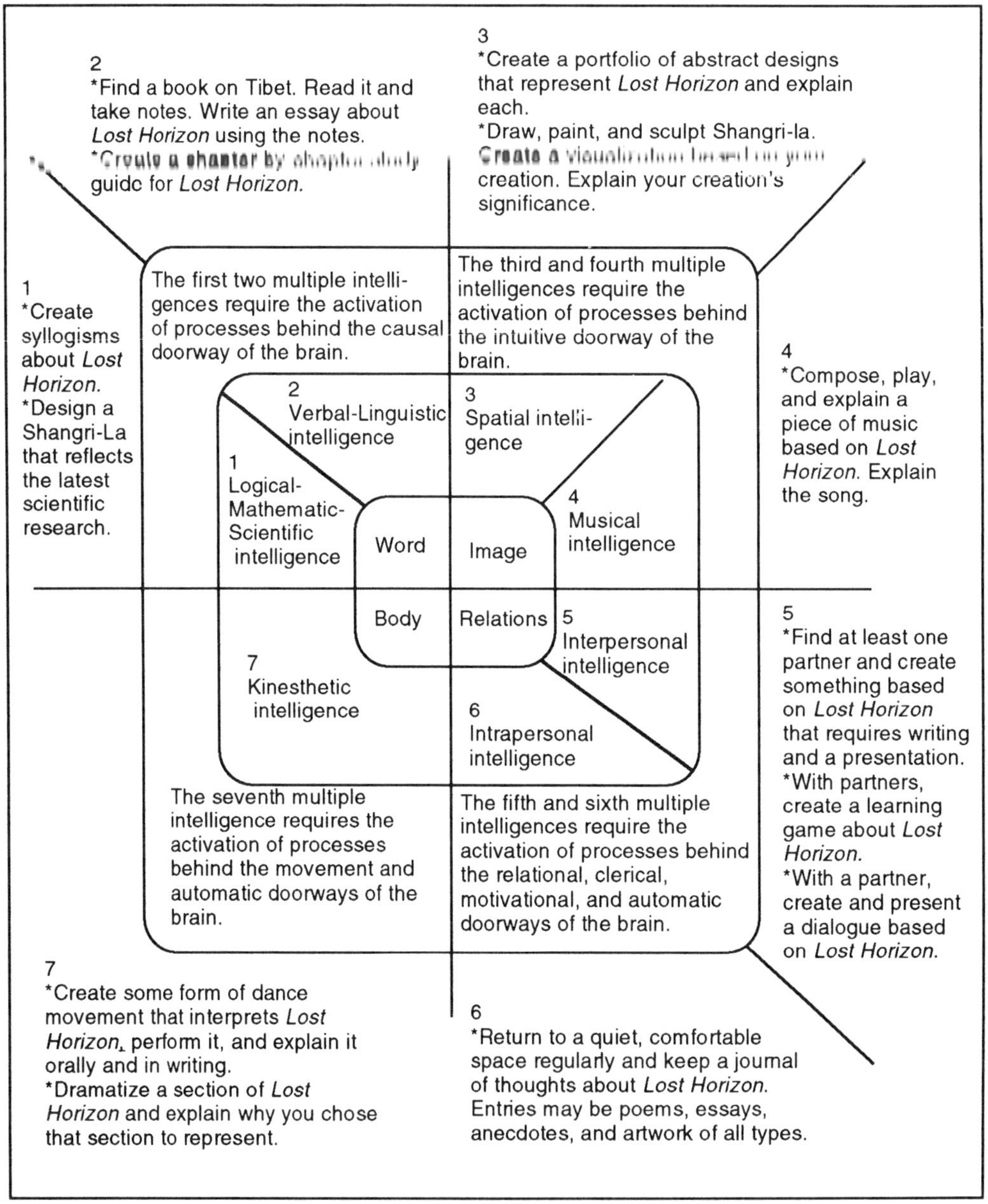


Figure 9.2. The *Lost Horizon* project using the integrated model of the 7 Doorways of the brain and the theory of multiple intelligences

# 10. THE DOORWAYS TO SCHOOL REFORM AND RESTRUCTURE

*Inspiration, hunger: these are the qualities that drive good schools. The best we educational planners can do is to create the most likely conditions for them to flourish, and then get out of the way.*

—Theodore Sizer, *Horace's Compromise*

All this talk about models of learning and teaching is nice, but just look around at what really is. There are so many more examples of ho-hum, business-as-usual classrooms than of any that incorporate across-the-board generic and radical change. But change *is* taking place, some painstakingly slow and some overnight, right under our noses.

## Individuals

Within systems where the pace is slow there are individual teachers who are making a difference. They are offering opportunities to their lucky students, who must endure the systematic contrast between those classrooms and those where ho hum is still the rule. Yet even in the ho-hum classrooms there is a leavening taking place, a kind of influence and power that is contagious, especially when teachers witness what is going on in other classrooms and find themselves facing the next class, the next day, the next month, the coming years of their professional lives. We hear more and more the echo of teachers who say that what they are doing needs to change. Teachers who are motivated by the personal and professional results of their own reforms and restructuring can never return to the ho hum. Impossible!

Social and cognitive changes brought on by the complexity of life have placed enormous pressures on schools. If schools do not change voluntarily they will be forced to do so or pass into oblivion. The forces of change are nudging even the most staid administrators to sigh with relief at the presence of teachers who are student centered and challenging and for whom children are motivated to learn. These teachers' students get involved in the excitement and rewards of education and schooling.

Realizing these forces exist does not mean I underestimate the power of lethargy and inertia-filled individuals who collectively retard change and often work tediously and quite actively against it. Marvin Cetron and Margaret Gayle (1991) state,

> The highest hurdle for radical reformers may be the attitudes and limited abilities of teachers themselves. In fact, though many teachers claim to want a more vigorous, effective educational system, we wonder how many would give up traditional classroom discipline and take on the challenge of keeping students productive in the unstructured debates of a Coalition school. And in a nation where many educators would flunk the final exams required of their students, how many possess the knowledge and thinking skills for the Paideia program's intellectually demanding Socratic style? The most serious obstacle to slowing the spread of these new teaching methods is the dearth of teachers capable of adapting them. (124–25)

In spite of the inertia they perceive in our school system, however, Cetron and Gayle project a positive picture of things to come: "Despite such problems, there seems no doubt that in the next decade or so, Paideia, the Coalition of Essential Schools, and the Key School will have an enormous influence on educators. Though comparatively few schools will adopt these programs whole, elements of each concept will filter into classrooms throughout the nation. As a result, academic performance should rise quickly, and dropout rates fall, in the years to come" (125). Certainly the individual teacher will deal with these reforms and, at some point, make a decision that will help form a critical mass; in the blink of an eye the revolution in education will be in full swing.

## The Paideia Proposal

More than one hundred schools have adopted Mortimer Adler's Paideia Proposal. The beauty of the proposal is that it is simple and, like so much that possesses the virtue of simplicity, it is transforming.

### One Track and Three Goals

Adler proposes heterogeneous grouping of grades K through 12. Three educational goals drive the curriculum: (1) to offer an experience that nurtures a lifetime of mental, moral, and spiritual growth; (2) to offer an experience that grooms students to participate actively and intelligently in our democracy throughout life; and (3) to offer an experience that helps students develop basic skills common to all work in a society whose jobs require intelligent people. Adler adds that these goals require an experience that is nonspecialized and nonvocationalized.

#### *Three Kinds of Knowledge, Three Teaching Styles*

According to the Paideia model, there are three kinds of knowledge that students acquire in different ways, so each requires a different teaching style. Students acquire organized knowledge by memorizing data; teachers must take a didactic, lecture-and-feedback approach to teach such knowledge. Students acquire learning skills by practicing and understanding; teachers must coach students and supervise opportunities for students to practice exercises that develop the students' learning skills. Students understand ideas and values by questioning and challenging answers to questions. Teachers can use Socratic questioning methods and active discussions to facilitate this learning. Because language, literature, the fine arts, mathematics, natural science, history, geography, social studies, and foreign language offer opportunities in the three types of knowledge, these courses comprise the core curriculum in Paideia schools.

### *7 Doorways Model into Paideia*

Figure 10.1 illustrates how the Paideia approach incorporates the 7 doorways.

- Organized knowledge and the didactic teaching approach are behind Doorway 1, causation, and Doorway 5, administration.
- Skills of learning and their concomitant coaching requirements involve Doorway 1, causation. Behind this door students calculate,

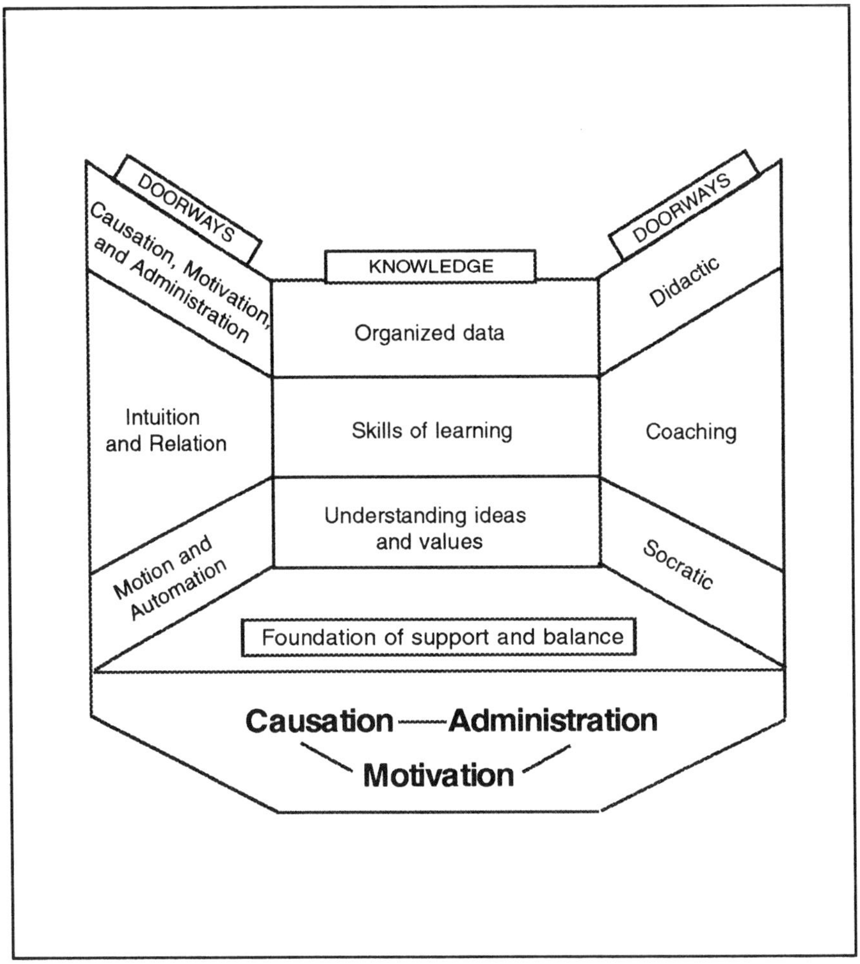


Figure 10.1. Paideia and the 7 Doorways model

measure, and think in sequential, systematic ways. When the core activities require imagination and nonlinear creativity, students can call Doorway 2, intuition, into play. This area of knowledge also requires teachers to emphasize Doorway 4, relation, because the interaction is more one-on-one.

- The understanding of ideas and values opens all the doorways, including Doorway 7, motion, because artistic activities, especially drama, require movement. Since this area of knowledge is artistic, creative, and movement oriented, it calls also for the proprioceptive awareness behind Doorway 3, automation.

The organized and purposeful structure that characterizes the Paideia Proposal gives it qualities important to the world of Doorways 5 and 6. The Paideia Proposal asks teachers and students to open all 7 Doorways of whole-brain learning with a slight emphasis on Doorways 1, 5, and 6.

For more information about the Paideia Proposal, write Skyline High School, Oakland Unified School District, 1025 Second Ave., Oakland, CA 94606, or call (415) 836-8200.

## The Coalition of Essential Schools and 7 Doorways Model

Theodore R. Sizer's book *Horace's Compromise: The Dilemma of the American High School* became the seed that grew into a reform movement, the Coalition of Essential Schools. At present there are more than one hundred that are full-fledged members and a host of others waiting to belong.

The basic structure includes units of not more than five hundred students. Teacher-to-student ratios are 1 to 80. The curriculum is concentrated, deep but not broad, and the governing principle is "less is more." Teachers plan together, schedules are flexible, and students display their competency and expertise in exhibitions.

### *The Common Principles of Coalition Schools and the 7 Doorways model*

There are nine principles that guide the schools in the coalition (see figure 10.2):

1. *Minds are to be well used.* To use them well requires experiences in all the doorways.

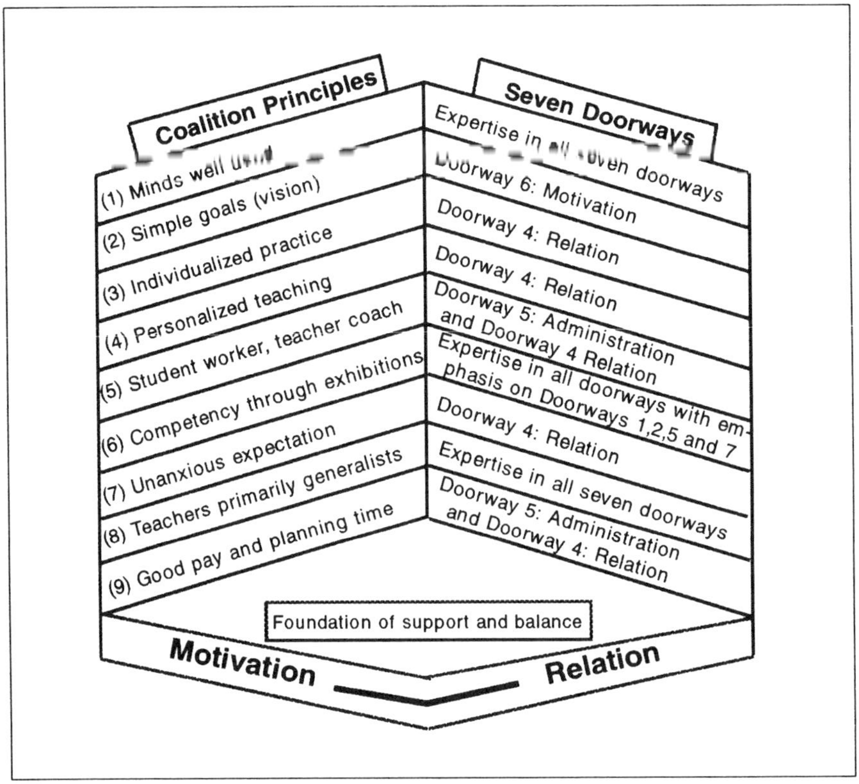


Figure 10.2. Coalition and the 7 Doorways model

2. *Goals should be simple but powerful.* Because of the coalition's vision and the focus it elicits from its membership, Doorway 6 embraces all that the coalition does every day.
3. *While goals apply to all students, students reach these goals individually.* Because the structure allows and demands a person-to-person, teacher-to-student approach, the overall curriculum recognizes the necessity of Doorway 4 (relations).
4. *Personalized teaching is necessary.* This principle emphasizes Doorway 4 as well.
5. *The idea that the student is a worker and the teacher a coach is central to methodology.* Because the curriculum is ordered around this principle and because coaching participates in the personal approach to teaching, Doorways 4 and 5 are important.

6. *Students must show competency by displaying their work in exhibitions.* Because this approach emphasizes the experience of what students create, all 7 Doorways are important. There is an emphasis on order and organization.
7. *A tone of unanxious expectation should permeate the school.* Creating a challenging environment of cooperation emphasizes Doorway 4 realities.
8. *The teaching staff should be generalists first and specialists second.* One of the major goals of the coalition schools is to emancipate the overall potentials of students without forcing them into specialized categories. Because of this generalist approach to content, coalition teachers must use all 7 Doorways.
9. *Teachers must be paid well and given time for planning.* The overall structure of excellence, collaboration, and planning means that Doorway 5 takes on the quality of collegiality in which all share a vested interest in the whole school.

To get the flavor of the dynamic marriage between Doorway 4 and Doorway 5 in coalition schools, I have included the example of Thayer High School in Winchester, New Hampshire, operated under the guidance of Dennis Littky. It is one of the brightest lights in the coalition movement. The November 1991 issue of the coalition newsletter, *Horace,* describes Littky's approach:

> Its principal, Dennis Littky, promotes teacher-talk with unflagging energy and a seemingly endless stream of strategies. Every Friday Littky's T.G.I.F. memo is required faculty reading, an exuberant amalgam of his reflections and questions, copies of provocative articles, lists of the subjects and times of the next week's meetings, and other diverse items. Two years ago, Littky passed out "those hardbound journals with pretty covers" to his staff in which they could correspond with him weekly about anything they chose ("I find out things they'd never say in person," he says). He circulates a videotape interviewing each teaching team for five minutes on this progress; he operates a consulting stable of Thayer teachers who are hired to travel and lecture, he brainstorms with teams on new strategies for parent involvement. (3)

*Horace* shows clearly that the coalition's emphasis on conversation, dialogue, and involvement requires Doorway 4.

For more information about the Coalition of Essential Schools, write Thayer High School, Winchester, NH 03470, or call (603) 239-8904.

## The Key School

Located in Indianapolis, Indiana, the Key School for grades K through 6 used Howard Gardner's theory of multiple intelligences and Mihaly Csikszentmihalyi's theory of flow states to restructure their school. Parent-advisor groups, presence of the community in classrooms, day care, and longer days for special programs form the atmosphere of the school.

At its core, the curriculum provides a balance between Gardner's seven intelligences and time for games that help students get into flow states that transfer to other academic areas. Mihaly Csikszentmihalyi (1990) coined the term "flow states" or "optimal experience states" to refer to times when "attention can be freely invested to achieve a person's goals, because there is no disorder to straighten out, no threat for the self to defend against" (40).

Flow states result in joy, self-control, and a sense of timelessness. Students are entranced by what they are doing, and their focus allows the brain to go in and out of alpha. Such freedom releases new feelings, new thoughts, and new associations, and certainly contributes to the overall motivation to continue learning, doing, and being.

Bruce Campbell (1991) also uses Gardner's intelligences in the classroom. Campbell describes how he restructured his third-grade class in Marysville, Washington: "I organized my third grade classroom into seven learning centers, each dedicated to one of the 7 intelligences. The students spend approximately 2/3 of each day moving through the centers—15 to 20 minutes at each center. Curriculum is thematic and the centers provide seven different ways for the students to learn the subject matter" (12).

Note that people have different interpretations of how to use the seven intelligences. The idea is to value each intelligence and to give students a variety of opportunities to learn. Students do not have to become competent in all intelligences—some will always be stronger in expressing themselves through dance, for example, than through writing.

For more information about the Key School, write Key School, Indianapolis Public Schools, 1401 E. 10th St., Indianapolis, IN 46201, or call (317) 226-4297.

## An Activity by Which to Part Company

### The Last Step

Time: Midmorning, late May
Place: Emerson School, Fitzwilliam, New Hampshire
Weather: Sunny and dry
General description of the day: As the sun passes through tall grass that casts shadows on a stone wall, it is gently painting individual stones. Stillness prevails.
The students: Fifth graders
The activity: Ten minutes to sit alone before this natural wonder, to draw it, and to respond briefly to the kind of clarity the experience gives
The drawings: They prove to be sensitive, filled with perspective, refined, and delicate.
The writing: Here they are, fifth graders at their best behind Doorway 2:

> When I was looking at those rocks I saw that life is not just sports. —Arlis

> It felt like I could do everything. It felt like I could draw everything there would be.—Carl

> It felt good because I was free and I didn't have to make one decision the whole time. It was peaceful and joyful.—Keith

> I felt clear when everything was still and I was relaxed and the leaves were rustling.—Brian

> I felt interested on how it would turn out. I thought it was interesting how the different textures and shapes and colors made a difference. —Ruth

> I felt that there's really no right way to draw the rocks but only to draw what you think.—Luke

> Being clear in your life is a neat feeling for me. It is like nothing matters and you're so carefree. Everything is still and you can think clearly. Now I know how Joanna felt.—Sarah
>
> How I got clear is I stared at the stone wall for a minute or so and my mind went off on thinking about drawing the stone wall.—Monika
>
> I think getting clear within yourself is like letting your mind just zoom off and not thinking about other things, just focus on what you're doing.—Elizabeth
>
> I thought that it was neat. Because that was the first time that I had done that before. I felt too that I was an artist and I've done it before but I hadn't.—Beth
>
> I think it was weird. It felt like I was really Joanna and I was a painter. —Margaret
>
> I felt very relaxed.—Ryan

## The Preceding Steps

The previous section describes the culminating activity of a project based on May Sarton's *Joanna and Ulysses*. Following is the rest of the project:

1. Read *Joanna and Ulysses,* discussing the themes and ideas while you do so.
2. Discuss, paraphrase, and illustrate the following quotations from the book:
    - "It was a perfect morning world, the sea soft and silken blue and the sky still flushed with rose."
    - "Because if I can see these stones and this tuft of grass with absolute clarity for itself alone, I somehow feel clear in myself."
    - "A woman alone and who seems happy to be alone arouses mixed emotions . . . "

The second passage is the basis for the last step described earlier.

3. Choose words from the book and have students use them to write two paragraphs that describe the story.

4. Have the students arrange ten illustrations from the book in sequence and then explain their arrangements as a plot summary.

## The Teacher, the Students, and Doorway 2

The teacher, Theresa Majoy, did not plan the final step of this activity initially. She arrived at school one morning and was suddenly astounded by the experience of sunshine casting shadows of blades of grass upon the rocks. It occurred to her immediately that this was one of those magic moments her class could share. Intuition led to a plan that opened many fifth-grade Doorway 2s.

The best teachers are like this: they have an awareness and an openness to possibilities. They take advantage of those moments when everything seems to come together, when we see the connection between things and we are moved to another level of learning and teaching.

# BIBLIOGRAPHY


Adler, Mortimer. *The Paideia Proposal.* New York: Macmillan, 1982.

Angeles, Peter A. *The Dictionary of Philosophy.* New York: Harper and Row, 1981.

Arendt, Hannah. *The Life of the Mind.* Vol. 1, *Thinking.* New York: Harcourt Brace Jovanovich, 1978.

Augarde, Tony. *The Oxford Dictionary of Modern Quotations.* Oxford: Oxford University Press, 1991.

Baker, Rob. "The Dance of Libra." *Parabola* 16 (1991): 20–27.

Balaskas, Arthur. "Body Awareness." In *How Does It Feel: Exploring the World of the Senses,* edited by Mike Csaky. New York: Harmony, 1979.

Bateson, Gregory. *Mind and Nature: A Necessary Unity.* New York: Dutton, 1979.

Benzwie, Teresa. *A Moving Experience: Dance for Lovers of Children and the Child Within.* Tucson, Ariz.: Zephyr Press, 1988.

———. *A Moving Experience: The Video.* Can be used effectively with *A Moving Experience.* Tucson, Ariz.: Zephyr Press, 1981.

Berlyne, Daniel Ellis. *The Encyclopedia of Education.* s.v. "motivation." New York: Macmillan, Free Press, 1971.

Berman, Morris. *The Reenchantment of the World.* New York: Bantam, 1984.

Bettelheim, Bruno. *The Uses of Enchantment: The Meaning and Importance of Fairy Tales.* New York: Vintage, 1977.

Block, Peter. *The Empowered Manager: Positive Political Skills at Work.* San Francisco: Jossey Bass, 1987.

Bloom, Allan. *The Closing of the American Mind.* New York: Simon and Schuster, 1987.

*The Brain Kit.* Model and activities. Dominguez Hills, Calif.: Educational Insights.

Bruchac, Joseph, and Michael J. Caduto. *Keepers of the Earth: Native American Stories and Environmental Activities for Children.* Golden, Colo.: Fulcrum, 1988.

Bruner, Jerome S. *On Knowing: Essays for the Left Hand.* Cambridge: Harvard University Press, 1979.

Buscaglia, Leo. *The Fall of Freddy the Leaf.* New York: Holt, Rinehart and Winston, 1982.

Caine, Geoffrey, and Renata Nummela Caine. *Teaching and the Human Brain.* Alexandria, Va.: ASCD, 1991.

Campbell, Bruce. "Multiple Intelligence in the Classroom." *In Context* 27 (1991): 12–15.

Campbell, Don G. *Music: Physician for Times to Come.* Wheaton, Colo.: Quest Books, 1991.

———. *100 Ways to Improve Teaching Using Your Voice and Music: Pathways to Accelerate Learning.* Tucson, Ariz.: Zephyr Press, 1992.

———. *Sound Pathways: Using Your Voice and Music to Accelerate Learning.* Tape to accompany *100 Ways to Improve Teaching Using Your Voice and Music.* Tucson, Ariz.: Zephyr Press, 1992.

Campbell, Don G., and Chris Boyd Brewer. *Rhythms of Learning:* Tucson, Ariz: Zephyr Press, 1991.

Cetron, Marvin, and Margaret Gayle. *Educational Renaissance: Our Schools at the Turn of the 21st Century.* New York: St. Martin's, 1991.

Chall, J., and A. Mursky. *Education and the Brain: The Seventieth Yearbook of the National Society for the Study of Education, Part II.* Chicago: University of Chicago Press, 1978.

Cherry, Clare, Douglass Godwin, and Jesse Staples. *Is the Left Brain Always Right?* Belmont, Calif.: David S. Lake, 1989.

Clark, Barbara. *Growing Up Gifted.* Columbus, Ohio: Merrill, 1983.

Corneau, Guy. *Absent Fathers, Lost Sons.* Boston: Shambhala, 1991.

Cornell, Judith. *Drawing the Light from Within.* New York: Prentice Hall, 1990.

Csikszentmihalyi, Mihaly. *Flow: The Psychology of Optimal Experiences.* New York: Harper and Row, 1990.

Delza, Sophia. *T'ai-Chi Ch'iian: Body and Mind in Harmony.* New York: Suny Press, 1961.

Dewey, John. *Experience and Education.* New York: Collier Books, 1963.

Diamond, Marian. *Enriching Heredity: The Impact of the Environment on the Anatomy of the Brain.* New York: Macmillan, Free Press, 1988.

Eccles, Sir John, and Daniel N. Robinson. *The Wonder of Being Human: Our Brain and Our Mind.* New York: Macmillan, Free Press, 1984.

Eppig, Peter, Wendy Knowles, and Peter Monether. *The Critical Skills Classroom.* Keene, N.H.: Antioch-New England Graduate School, 1989.

Ferguson, Marilyn. *The Aquarian Conspiracy: Personal and Social Transformation in the 1980s.* Los Angeles: Jeremy P. Tarcher, 1980.

Flaste, Richard. "Sidelined by Loneliness." *The Boston Globe Magazine* (April 28, 1991): 14–15, 26–27.

Fuller, R. Buckminster. *On Education.* Amherst: W. Mass Press, 1979.

Galyean, Beverly-Colleene. *Mind Sight: Learning through Imagery.* Long Beach, Calif.: Center for Integrative Learning, 1983.

Gardner, Howard. *Frames of Mind: The Theory of Multiple Intelligence.* New York: Basic Books, 1985.

Garner, Philip. *Rube Goldberg: A Retrospective.* New York: Delilah Communications, 1983.

Garvey, Catherine. *Play.* Cambridge: Harvard University Press, 1977.

Gawain, Shakti. *Creative Visualization.* New York: Bantam Books, 1982.

Gazzaniga, Michael. *Mind Matters: How the Mind and Brain Interact to Create Our Conscious Lives.* Boston: Houghton Mifflin, 1988.

———. *The Social Brain: Discovering the Networks of the Mind.* New York: Basic Books, 1985.

Gilligan, Carol. *In a Different Voice: Psychological Theory and Women's Development.* Cambridge: Harvard University Press, 1983.

Gilligan, Carol, Nona P. Lyons, and Trudy J. Hammer. *Making Connections: The Relational Worlds of Adolescent Girls at Emma Willard School.* Cambridge: Harvard University Press, 1990.

Gilman, Robert. "The Trouble with Men." *In Context* 16 (Spring 1987): 5–9.

Glasser, William, *Control Theory in the Classroom.* New York: Harper and Row, 1986.

Goldberg, Philip. *The Intuitive Edge: Understanding and Developing Intuition.* Los Angeles: Jeremy P. Tarcher, 1983.

Goleman, Daniel, Paul Kaufman, and Ray Michael. *The Creative Spirit.* New York: E. P. Dutton, 1992.

Goode, Caron B., and Joy Lehni Watson. *The Mind Fitness Program for Esteem and Excellence: Guided Stories for Imagery in Whole-Brain Learning.* Tucson, Ariz.: Zephyr Press, 1992.

———. *Reaching the Star Within.* Tape to accompany *The Mind Fitness Program.* Tucson, Ariz.: Zephyr Press, 1992.

Gowan, John Curtis. *Development of the Psychedelic Individual.* Buffalo, N.Y.: State University College, 1974.

Granger, Bill, and Lori Granger. *The Magic Feather.* New York: Dell, 1989.

Gray, William, and Paul La Violette. *Brain-Mind Bulletin.* Theme Pack 15, 7–8.

Greene, Maxine. *The Dialectic of Freedom.* New York: Teacher's College Press, 1988.

———. *Landscapes of Learning.* New York: Teacher's College Press, 1978.

Grimm, Jacob, and Wilhelm Grimm. *Grimm's Fairy Tales.* London: Routledge and Kegan Paul, 1948.

Griscom, Chris. *Ocean Born.* Galisteo, New Mexico: The Light Institute, 1989.

Harrison, Alton, Jr., and Diane Musial. *Other Ways, Other Means: Altered Awareness Activities for Receptive Learning.* Santa Monica, Calif.: Goodyear Publishing, 1978.

Hart, Leslie. *Human Brain and Human Learning.* Oak Creek, Ariz.: Books for Educators, 1983.

Hart, Mickey, and Frederic Lieberman. *Planet Drum.* New York: Harper Collins, 1991.

Healy, Jane M. *Endangered Minds: Why Children Don't Think and What We Can Do about It.* New York: Simon and Schuster, 1990.

———. *Your Child's Growing Mind: A Parent's Guide to Learning from Birth to Adolescence.* New York: Doubleday, 1987.

Holt, John. *Freedom and Beyond.* New York: E. P. Dutton, 1972.

*Horace.* Coalition newsletter. Nov. 1991.

Houston, Jean. *The Possible Human: A Course in Extending Your Physical, Mental, and Creative Abilities.* Los Angeles: Jeremy P. Tarcher, 1982.

Hunt, Morton. *The Universe Within.* New York: Simon and Schuster, 1982.

Hutchinson, Michael. *Megabrain.* New York: Ballantine Books, 1986.

Jessell, David, and Anne Moir. *Brain Sex: The Real Difference between Men and Women.* New York: Dell, 1991.

Johnston, Charles M. *The Creative Imperative: A Four-Dimensional Theory of Human Growth and Planetary Evolution*. Berkeley, Calif.: Celestial Arts, 1984, 1986.

Jung, Carl. *Mandala Symbolism*. Princeton, N.J.: Princeton University Press, 1969.

Kahn, Robert D., and Peter H. Wapehal. *R. Buchminster Fuller on Education*. Amherst, Mass.: The University of Massachusetts Press, 1979.

Keen, Sam. *Fire in the Belly*. New York: Bantam Books, 1991.

Kessler, Shelly. "Teaching Presence." *Holistic Education Review* 4 (1991): 4–5.

Kidder, Tracy. *Among Schoolchildren*. Boston: Houghton Mifflin, 1989.

Kohl, Herbert. *Basic Skills*. New York: Bantam Books, 1982.

———. *Growing Minds: On Becoming a Teacher*. New York: Harper and Row, 1984.

———. *I Won't Learn from You!* Minneapolis: Milkweed Editions, 1991.

Kohn, Alfie. *No Contest: The Case against Competition*. Boston: Houghton Mifflin, 1986.

Konner, Melvin. *The Tangled Wing*. New York: Holt, Rinehart and Winston, 1982.

LaMeres, Clare. *The Winner's Circle: Yes, I Can*. Newport Beach, Calif. LaMeres Lifestyles Unlimited, 1990.

Lawrence, Gordon. *People Types and Tiger Stripes*. Gainesville, Fla.: Center for Application of Psychological Type, 1984.

Lazear, David. *Seven Ways of Knowing: Understanding Multiple Intelligences*. 2d ed. Palatine, Ill.: Skylight Publishing, 1991.

———. *Seven Ways of Teaching: The Artistry of Teaching with Multiple Intelligences*. Palatine, Ill.: Skylight Publishing, 1991.

Leonard, George B. *Education and Ecstasy and the Great School Reform Hoax*. New York: Delacorte Press, 1968.

Lipman, Mathew, Fredrick S. Oscanyan, and Ann Margaret Sharp. *Philosophical Inquiry: An Instruction Manual to Accompany Harry Stottlemeier's Discovery*. 2d ed. New York: University Press of America, 1984.

Lipman, Mathew, and Ann Margaret Sharp. *Ethical Inquiry: Instructional Manual to Accompany Lisa*. New York: University Press of America, 1985.

Loye, David. *The Sphinx and the Rainbow: Brain, Mind, and Future Vision.* Boulder: Shambhala, 1983.

McCarthy, Bernice. *The 4MAT System: Teaching to Learning Styles with Right/Left Mode Techniques.* Rev. ed. Barrington, Ill.: Excel, 1987.

McKenzie, Jamieson. "The New Agenda." *High School Instructor* Spring 1989.

MacLean, Paul D. *A Triune Concept of Brain and Behavior.* Toronto: Toronto University Press, 1973.

Margulies, Nancy, *Mapping Inner Space.* Tucson, Ariz.: Zephyr Press, 1991.

Mason, Kathy. *Going Beyond Words: The Art and Practice of Visual Thinking.* Tucson, Ariz.: Zephyr Press, 1991.

Mathews, Gareth. *Philosophy and the Young Child.* Cambridge: Harvard University Press, 1980.

Miller, Alice. *The Drama of the Gifted Child.* New York: Basic Books, 1987.

Montessori, Maria. *The Secret of Childhood.* New York: Ballantine Books, 1966.

Morris, Susan, and Bernice McCarthy. *4MAT in Action II: Sample Lesson Plans for Use with the 4MAT System.* Barrington, Ill.: Excel, 1990.

"Movement Psychology Freeing 'Postural Beliefs.'" *Brain-Mind Bulletin* 8 (1983): 1–2.

Murdock, Maureen. *Spinning Inward: Using Guided Imagery with Children.* Boston: Shambhala, 1987.

Ornstein, Robert, and David Sobel. *The Healing Brain: Breakthrough Medical Discoveries about How the Brain Keeps Us Healthy.* New York: Simon and Schuster, 1987.

Pearce, Joseph Chilton. *Evolution's End: Claiming the Potential of Our Inheritance.* San Francisco: Harper San Francisco, HarperCollins, 1992.

———. *Magical Child Matures.* New York: E. P. Dutton, 1985.

Phenix, Philip H. *Realms of Meaning: A Prospective through Retrospective.* New York: McGraw Hill, 1964.

Poe, Edgar Allen. *The Works of Edgar Allan Poe.* Vol. 9. New York: Funk and Wagnall, 1904.

Prigogine, Ilya. *Order Out of Chaos: Man's New Dialogue with Nature.* Toronto: Bantam Books, 1984.

Restak, Richard. *The Brain.* New York: Bantam Books, 1984.

Russell, Bertrand. *Our Knowledge of the External World.* New York: Mentor Books, 1960.

Sarton, May. *Joanna and Ulysses.* New York: Norton, 1987.

Shelley, Mary. *Frankenstein.* New York: E. P. Dutton, 1965.

Silverstein, Shel. *The Giving Tree.* New York: Harper and Row, 1988.

Simon, Tobin, and Linda Trechter-Metcalf. *Proprioceptive Writing Center Bulletin.*

Sizer, Theodore R. *Horace's Compromise: The Dilemma of the American High School.* Boston: Houghton Mifflin, 1984.

Steinem, Gloria. *Revolution from Within: A Book of Self-Esteem.* Boston: Little, Brown, 1992.

Talbot, Michael. *The Holographic Universe.* New York: Harper Collins, 1991.

Van Dusen, Wilson. *The Natural Depth in Man.* New York: Swedenborg Foundation, 1972.

Vaughan, Frances E. *Awakening Intuition.* New York: Anchor Books, 1979.

Webb, Terry Tyler. *Accelerated Learning with Music: A Trainer's Manual.* Norcross, Ga.: Accelerated Learning Systems, 1990.

Wharton, William P. "Imagery and Readability of Textbooks." In *Imagery in Education,* edited by Anees A. Sheikh and Katharina S. Sheikh. Amityville, N.Y.: Baywood, 1985, 145–60.

Williams, Linda Verlee. *Teaching for the Two Sided Mind: A Guide to Right-Brain–Left-Brain Education.* New York: Simon and Schuster, 1983.

Wolf, Fred Alan. *Taking the Quantum Leap: The New Physics for Nonscientists.* San Francisco: Harper and Row, 1981.

# COPYRIGHT ACKNOWLEDGMENTS

*The Reenchantment of the World* by Morris Bermon, © 1981 by Morris Bermon, used by permission of the publisher, Cornell University Press.

*The Empowered Manager: Positive Political Skills at Work* by Peter Block, p. 132, © 1987 by Peter Block and Jossey-Bass Inc., publishers.

*The Closing of the American Mind* by Allan Bloom, © 1987 by Allan Bloom, reprinted by permission of Simon & Schuster, Inc.

*The Spiritual Life of Children* by Robert Coles, © 1990 by Robert Coles, reprinted by permission of Houghton Mifflin Co. All rights reserved.

*Creative Visualization* by Shakti Gawain, copyright 1978, reprinted with permission of New World Library, San Rafael, Calif. 94903.

*The Intuitive Edge* by Philip Goldberg, © 1983 by Philip Goldberg, Los Angeles: Jeremy P. Tarcher, Inc., 1983.

*The Creative Spirit* by Dan Goleman, Paul Kaufman, and Michael Ray, © 1992 by Alvin H. Perlmutter, Inc., used by permission of the publisher, Dutton, an imprint of New American Library, a division of Penguin Books USA Inc.

*Dialectic of Freedom,* (New York: Teachers College Press, © 1988 by Teachers College, Columbia Universiy, all rights reserved), pp. 20–21, reprinted by permission of the publisher.

*In Context: A Quarterly of Humane Sustainable Culture,* subscriptions $24/yr, single issues $6, P.O. Box 11470, Bainbridge Island, Wash. 98110.

*Among Schoolchildren* by Tracy Kidder, © 1989 by John Tracy Kidder, reprinted by permission of Houghton Mifflin Co. All rights reserved.

*The Drama of the Gifted Child* by Alice Miller, translated by Ruth Ward, © 1981 by Basic Books, Inc., © 1979 Suhrkamp Verlag Frankfurt am Main, reprinted by permission of BasicBooks, a division of HarperCollins Publishers Inc.

*Spinning Inward,* by Maureen Murdock, © 1987 by Maureen Murdock, reprinted by arrangement with Shambhala Publications, Inc., 300 Massachusetts Ave., Boston, Mass. 02115.

*The Healing Brain* by Robert Ornstein and David Sobel, © 1987 by The Institute for the Study of Human Knowledge, reprinted by permission of Simon & Schuster, Inc.

*Parabola: The Magazine of Myth and Tradition,* vol. 16, no. 4, (Winter, 1991), subscription $20/year (4 issues), back issues $8 from *Parabola,* 656 Broadway, New York, N.Y. 10012.

*Teaching for the Two Sided Mind: A Guide to Right-Brain, Left-Brain Education,* © 1983 by Linda Verlee Williams, reprinted by permission of Simon & Schuster, Inc.

# INDEX

# Additional Resources from Zephyr Press

SEVEN PATHWAYS OF LEARNING

**Teaching Students and Parents about Multiple Intelligences**

by David Lazear

David Lazear dedicates his new book to helping students tap into their full learning potential.

Encourage your students to pass through four distinct levels of thinking about intelligence. Each step encompasses a wider spiral of understanding. Make effective use of the seven intelligences by going through these levels—

- Tacit—becoming aware of individual capabilities
- Aware—strengthening personal intelligence
- Strategic—knowing how and when to use each type of intelligence
- Reflective—integrating multiple intelligences into everyday life

Incorporate thinking about intelligences into your classroom. Show students how to master classroom assignments and to enrich lifelong learning.

For teachers of K-Adult.
302 pages, 8 1/2" x 11", softbound.

ZB45-W—$30

To order, write or call—
Zephyr Press
P.O. Box 13448-W
Tucson, Arizona 85732
Phone—(602) 322-5090
FAX—(602) 323-9402

You can also request a free copy of our current catalog showing other learning materials that foster whole-brain learning, creative thinking, and self-awareness.

MAPPING INNER SPACE

**Learning and Teaching Mind Mapping**

by Nancy Margulies

Mind mapping is a significant advance over traditional, linear note taking. Use mind mapping for personal note taking, in curriculum planning, in group process in the classroom, and as a teaching strategy in daily lessons.

Using a mind map, you can record more information on a page and show relationships among various concepts.

Mind mapping integrates the processes of both sides of the brain—the linear left side and the global right side.

ZB18W . . . $24.95

RHYTHMS OF LEARNING

**Creative Tools for Developing Lifelong Skills**

by Don G. Campbell & Chris Boyd Brewer

Learn about the physical and emotional highs and lows to promote a learning environment that is less stressful and more focused. Specific activities for teachers precede and complement the student activities.

- Discover the best learning modes of your students
- Learn to use music, art, movement, and drama to promote optimal learning states
- Use effective rhythms of presentation in your teaching
- Learn about and use the methods of Lozanov and Tomatis and the techniques of accelerated learning

**Grades K-Adult.**

ZB21W . . . $24.95